DISCARDED BY

MACPHÁIDÍN LIBRARY

CUSHING-MARTIN LIBRARY
STONEHILL COLLEGE
NORTH EASTON, MASSACHUSETTS 02356

Language Disorders in Children

Recent Advances

Editor in chief, Speech, Language, and Hearing Disorders Series
William H. Perkins, PhD

Language Disorders in Children

Recent Advances

edited by
Audrey L. Holland, PhD
Speech and Hearing Center
University of Pittsburgh

College-Hill Press, San Diego, California

College-Hill Press
4284 41st Street
San Diego, California 92105

© 1984 by College-Hill Press, Inc.

All rights, including that of translation, reserved. No part of this publication may be reproduced, stored in a retrieval system, or transmitted in any form or by any means, electronic, mechanical, recording, or otherwise, without the prior written permission of the publisher.

Library of Congress Cataloging in Publication Data

Main entry under title:
Language disorders in children.

  Bibliography: p.
  Includes indexes.
  1. Language disorders in children. I. Holland, Audrey L.
[DNLM: 1. Language disorders--In infancy and childhood. WL 340 L28757]
RJ496.L35L362 1983   618.92'855   83-7727
ISBN 0-933014-92-9

Printed in the United States of America

Publisher's Note

These volumes were developed under the supervision of a group of leading scientists charged with the responsibility of assessing the most critical book needs of the speech-language-hearing profession. In consultation with William H. Perkins and Raymond G. Daniloff, serving as editors in chief of the ensuing volumes on speech, language, and hearing disorders (Perkins) and speech, language, and hearing science (Daniloff), the publisher planned a series of nine mutually independent texts covering the entirety of state-of-the-art knowledge in these disciplines, with contributions by respected, productive, and current scholars known for their expertise as specialists in key areas.

Each contribution has been stringently refereed for content, pedagogy, and practical value for students and practitioners by the individual volume editors, Charles Berlin, Janis Costello, Raymond Daniloff, Audrey Holland, James Jerger, Rita Naremore, and their designated reviewers, in close consultation throughout with the editors in chief and the publisher. Users are thus assured that their needs for accurate, timely information, reflecting the highest standards of scholarship and professionalism, have been faithfully met.

On behalf of the speech-language-hearing profession, its researchers, teachers, practitioners, and students, present and future, the publisher thanks the more than 100 authors and editors who have given generously of their time and knowledge to produce this magnificent contribution to the literature.

Language Disorders in Children, edited by Audrey Holland, is one of nine state-of-the-art volumes comprising the College-Hill Press series covering the current body of knowledge in speech, language, and hearing.

Volume Titles:	Editors:
Speech Disorders in Children	Janis Costello
Speech Disorders in Adults	Janis Costello
Speech Science	Raymond Daniloff
Language Disorders in Children	Audrey Holland
Language Disorders in Adults	Audrey Holland
Language Science	Rita Naremore
Pediatric Audiology	James Jerger
Hearing Disorders in Adults	James Jerger
Hearing Science	Charles Berlin
Editor in chief, Speech, Language, and Hearing Disorders Series:	William H. Perkins
Editor in chief, Speech, Language, and Hearing Science Series:	Raymond G. Daniloff

Contents

Contributors

Anthony S. Bashir, PhD
The Children's Hospital Medical
Center
Division of Hearing & Speech
300 Longwood Ave.
Boston, MA 02115

Thomas F. Campbell
Department of Speech Pathology
Glenrose Hospital
Edmonton, Alberta, Canada

Marie Capozzi, MA
Speech Pathology & Audiology
University of Pittsburgh
Pittsburgh, PA 15260

Robin S. Chapman, PhD
Department of Communicative
Disorders
University of Wisconsin–Madison
Madison, WI 53706

Laurence B. Leonard, PhD
Department of Audiology & Speech
Sciences
Purdue University
West Lafayette, IN 47907

Jacqueline Weis Liebergott, PhD
Emerson College
Division of Communication Disorders
168 Beacon St.
Boston, MA 02116

Jon F. Miller, PhD
Department of Communicative
Disorders
University of Wisconsin–Madison
Madison, WI 53706

Beth Mineo, MA
Speech Pathology & Audiology
University of Pittsburgh
Pittsburgh, PA 15260

Elizabeth M. Prather, PhD
Department of Speech &
Hearing Science
Arizona State University
Tempe, AZ 85287

Martin C. Schultz, PhD
The Children's Hospital Medical
Center
Division of Hearing & Speech
300 Longwood Ave.
Boston, MA 02115

Lynn S. Snyder, PhD
Department of Speech Pathology
and Audiology
University of Denver
Denver, CO 80208

Susan E. Weismer
Waisman Center on Mental
Retardation and Human
Development
University of Wisconsin–Madison
Madison, WI 53706

M. Jeanne Wilcox, PhD
Division of Speech Pathology and
Audiology
Kent State University
Kent, OH 44242

Foreword

From 1977 to 1982, while editing the *Journal of Speech and Hearing Disorders,* I became increasingly aware of the rate at which information about communication disorders was expanding. Not only was it an information explosion, it was a conceptual explosion as well, particularly in the area of children's language. We are departing rapidly from a relatively insular profession in which clinical practice has been based largely on what we could learn from our own experience. What we are moving toward is a theory-based profession in which we are open to broad-ranging conceptions, most notably from linguistics, medicine, and psychology.

It was against this background that *Recent Advances: Speech, Language, and Hearing Pathology* was spawned. In accepting the responsibility of being editor in chief, I saw several opportunities. Above all, it offered a vehicle by which the profession could remain current. Some areas have moved so rapidly that they bear little resemblance to what they were even a decade ago. Not only has information proliferated, but so have the journals and texts in which it has been preserved. Here, then, in *Recent Advances,* was an opportunity to organize a coherent and comprehensive account of the current state of affairs in all clinical aspects of speech, language, and hearing.

A price paid for advancement of knowledge is not only inability to consume the increasing glut, but even to comprehend it. One must almost be a specialist to understand what other specialists are talking about. To chronicle the state of the art across all areas of communication disorders, and still make responsible statements, would require the best minds available in each area. To know who the experts in these areas are, and to obtain their participation, would require scholars of such stature as to attract them. Hence, my most important responsibility in this project was the selection of volume editors. I take great pride that Janis Costello, Audrey Holland, and James Jerger agreed to participate.

With their respective editorships established, my remaining responsibility was to consult with them in determining the chapters needed to report the state of the art in their areas, and in selecting authors most qualified to prepare the chapters. We sought authors who not only are established scholars, but who also write with clarity. We were as concerned that anyone in the profession be able to read and understand what is going on in any area as we were with assembling the best information available. Aside from nudging the project along occasionally and final editing, I can claim little credit for the sterling quality of these texts. That credit belongs to the editors.

William H. Perkins
Editor in chief

Preface

I spend most of my professional energies in the study of adult language disorders, while maintaining an interest in child language disorders and their remediation. However, as knowledge in both areas has exploded, it has been increasingly impossible to keep in touch with changes and advances in the far larger, more often pacesetting area of child language. When I undertook to edit this volume, it was simultaneously a challenge and a wonderful opportunity to "catch up" on recent advances in child language. The trick, of course, was to choose the authors carefully and to learn from them as one occasionally reunited a split infinitive or knocked off an unintended redundancy. Because editing this book has been such a heady learning experience for me, and because it has allowed me to become relatively "caught up," I am very pleased to introduce *Language Disorders in Children* to its readers.

Laurence Leonard, who wrote his chapter while training for the Boston Marathon, initiates the volume with a thoughtful resume of the state of the art in the study of normal language acquisition. His chapter critically highlights recent developments, and carefully separates the significant from the merely trendy. He takes the important next step as well—relating advances in the general study of child language to their application to children with language disorders.

Following Leonard's chapter, Jacqueline Liebergott, Anthony Bashir, and Martin Schultz offer a new look at the knowns and unknowns about at-risk infants and their likelihood of developing speech and language disorders. Because the easy belief is that at-risk infants are at-risk for problems generally, the chapter may come as a surprise to a number of readers. The straightforwardness of its logic and clarity of its argument, however, cannot easily be dismissed. It is anticipated that this chapter will have great professional impact.

Three chapters next discuss children who have developmental disorders of language. An arbitrary editorial decision was made to split the population by age, into preschool children, school-age children, and adolescents. The preschool chapter by M. Jeanne Wilcox, and the school-age chapter by Lynn Snyder, relate meaningfully to each other and to Leonard's chapter, without sacrificing the important contrasts that necessarily differentiate diagnosis and treatment of language disorders in the two age groups. Wilcox' chapter not only sets the scholarly context for language remediation, but it provides a nuts-and-bolts application to treatment. Snyder's chapter offers an insightful analysis of the relationships between language and learning disorders, providing a model for subsequent study and clinical intervention as well.

Elizabeth Prather's chapter on language disorders in adolescents is a departure from the previous two, because the study of normal and disordered language lacks the interest and richness of data apparent in the study of preschoolers and school-age children. Prather's chapter is a crisp and pointed review of the little-studied area; but, its major focus must be seen as its plea for more information.

Children who acquire language disorders after a period of previously normal development are different in some substantial ways from children who have failed to develop language normally. However these differences are not well studied. In this volume's chapter on children with acquired seizure disorders, Jon Miller, Thomas Campbell, Robin Chapman, and Susan Weismer provide a germinal model for the study of children with acquired disorders of language. The work can serve as a model for other acquired language disorders in children, including such diverse problems as closed-head injury and sickle cell disease.

No matter how thoroughly trained the speech/language pathologist might be, if that training occurred 5 years or more ago, that training has failed to prepare for the present significant movement in nonvocal communication. Marie Capozzi and Beth Mineo provide readers with a thorough tutorial designed to acquaint them with the exploding and often confusing, field of augmentive communication and its accompanying technology. The comprehensive nature of their review should fill the void that exists for so many of us as a result of the recent rapid accumulation of techniques and instrumentation.

Rather than continue to preview the chapters in the book, it is important to let them talk for themselves. It has been very rewarding to work with these authors and to learn from them. I have no doubt that you will be similarly rewarded by what follows.

Audrey L. Holland
Editor

Laurence B. Leonard

Normal Language Acquisition: Some Recent Findings and Clinical Implications

For some time, speech-language clinicians have made considerable use of the available literature on normal language acquisition when devising assessment and treatment strategies for language-disordered children. This type of application is only as good as the source, however, and when new information is gained concerning the nature of language acquisition in normally developing children, aspects of adopted intervention strategies may need to be re-evaluated. It is appropriate, therefore, that a volume on recent advances in the study of language disorders also include a discussion of recent findings in the area of normal language acquisition.

The topics included in this chapter are those that seem to me to be both current and clinically applicable. In the interest of space, not all appropriate topics are represented. The final selection was based on the additional consideration that the chapter reflect findings covering a wide range of linguistic abilities acquired during childhood. These abilities are discussed more or less in developmental order.

As will be apparent in the chapters that follow, some of the findings reviewed here have served as the foundation for recent research with language-disordered children. In order to avoid duplication, this applied research will not be discussed. However, these studies are only just beginning to appear, and there are a number of clinical issues arising from the normal-language findings that have yet to be addressed. Some of these are noted at the end of each section of the chapter.

© College-Hill Press, Inc. All rights, including that of translation, reserved. No part of this publication may be reproduced without the written permission of the publisher.

Normal Language Acquisition: Some Recent Findings

Early Comprehension and Production

Early comprehension

One trend seen in the literature on normal language development during the past several years is an increased interest in young children's comprehension skills. From Huttenlocher's (1974) classic report of early language comprehension, we had reason to believe that children as young as nine months of age may respond appropriately to words and short phrases. However, children at this young age are not the most co-operative of subjects, and, thus, assessment of comprehension has had to rely on informal techniques.

Chapman (1978) has described some of the limitations to interpretation that can arise from the use of such informal procedures. She identified several comprehension strategies used by young children that can give the impression they understand more than they actually do. Some of these strategies are based on nonlinguistic cues and require no language comprehension. One such strategy is acting on objects that are noticed. Such a strategy might be seen in cases where an adult places an object in front of the child and says, "Pick up the X." Another nonlinguistic strategy is the imitation of the actions of others. For instance, the child may hold his arms up if, along with asking "Up?" the adult begins to reach for the child.

Other strategies may require lexical comprehension on the part of the child, but an uncritical assessment of the child's response may lead to the interpretation that he or she understands sentences. The strategy of doing what is usually done in the situation serves as a good example. For instance, when faced with an array consisting of a toy truck, brush, doll, and block, a child might respond correctly to the request, "Brush the dolly's hair," by comprehending the word "hair" and performing the usual action done with hair.

More recently, Oviatt (1980) has developed a method for assessing lexical comprehension in young children that allows one to draw more definitive conclusions concerning a child's comprehension ability than seems possible with most informal measures. This method is basically a training procedure. The child is provided with exposures to previously unknown object and action names. Following this exposure period, the child's comprehension of each word is tested. One important feature of this approach is that it allows one to compute the consistency of the child's response to the word relative to his or her response to a control word and his or her response when no word is provided.

Oviatt's (1980) procedure for assessing comprehension of an object name can serve as an illustration. A highly salient referent (a live rabbit or hamster housed in a transparent travel case) was placed to the side of the child. For three minutes the child was permitted to observe the animal, while the experimenter and the child's parent named it a total of 24 times. The child was then distracted with novel toys for the following three minutes. The experimenter then gained the child's attention and asked the child to locate the target referent ("Where's the rabbit?"), a nonexistent referent ("Where's the kawlow?"), and, in some cases, a familiar referent ("Where's the book?"") in alternating order. Instances where the child gazed back at the target referent constituted the measure of interest. Along with determining the rate of responding to the target and control questions, the frequency with which the child gazed back at the target referent when no question was asked was also considered, for purposes of determining a base rate. A child was credited with recognitory comprehension of the word if he or she showed no gazing responses to control questions and responded to the target questions at a rate that exceeded base rate. Oviatt found that on such tasks, recognitory comprehension seemed to show an abrupt emergence at approximately 10 to 11 months of age, and appeared very consistent by ages 12 to 14 months. Similar findings were seen for object and action names.

The clinical implications of the work of Chapman (1978) and Oviatt (1980) are substantial. With regard to the former, it seems that there are several factors unrelated to lexical comprehension per se that might allow a child to respond as if he or she understands the word being tested. Proper assessment of understanding of the word, then, would require elimination of these factors during testing. Requests for an action (e.g., "Wave bye-bye"), for example, should not be accompanied by behaviors the child can imitate, nor should they be made only when situational clues are available (e.g., "Go peek-a-boo," as the child is handed a blanket). Likewise, assessment of the child's comprehension of object names should include requests for objects when other objects are also present, and in situations in which the requested objects are not usually present (e.g., "Where's the ball?" requested at the snack table) as well as in situations in which they are.

It appears that the Oviatt (1980) procedure holds much promise for clinical application. The tasks currently available for assessing early lexical comprehension in language-disordered children require the child to perform acts such as retrieving or pointing to the correct referent from an array of objects, or performing, or making a doll perform, a requested action. Yet, young children just beginning to attach meanings to words

:ognitory comprehension of such words. Thus, if the
etermine a language-disordered child's readiness for com-
, Oviatt's procedure would seem to be most appropriate.
hown evidence of comprehending words and the clinical
⌐ ᴊ111ts to an assessment of the number of words comprehended, existing tasks might then be employed.

Word Production

Along with gaining a greater understanding of children's early lexical
comprehension, we have been able to form a clearer picture of their early
production of words. Much of the work devoted to word production has
focused on factors that influence a young child's tendency to use a particular word. One such factor is the phonological composition of the word.
For a number of years, diary and naturalistic studies of young children
have included the observation that many seem to avoid use of certain forms
of adult words (Ferguson, Peizer, & Weeks, 1973; Macken, 1976; Menn,
1976; Vihman, 1976). According to these accounts, a few lexical types are
selected that serve as the basis of the child's production system and attempts
at other kinds of lexical items are avoided. Interestingly, children seem to
vary in the particular adult forms selected and avoided. Some children have
primarily selected words with labial or apical consonants in the initial position (Leopold, 1947), others have selected words with word-initial velars
(Menn, 1971), and others have attempted words with word-initial fricatives
(Ferguson & Farwell, 1975). The initial consonant seems to serve as a
primary determiner in these cases (Shibamoto & Olmsted, 1978). However,
in some instances, children's selection and avoidance tendencies may involve
an interaction between the initial consonant and the syllable shape of words
(Macken, 1976).

One of the difficulties in interpreting reports of phonological selection
and avoidance tendencies in young children has been that there was no
way to rule out the possibility that they were not simply a reflection of
the differential frequencies of consonants and syllable shapes in the speech
heard in the child's environment. However, more recently, investigations
controlling for this frequency of exposure factor have appeared in the
literature. Schwartz and Leonard (1982) found that children with
expressive lexicons of approximately five words were more likely to
acquire the use of new words that contained consonants they had previously produced accurately than words containing consonants they had
shown no prior evidence of attempting, even when both types of words
had been exposed with equal frequency. Leonard, Schwartz, Morris, and

Chapman (1981) reported identical findings for children with expressive lexicons of approximately 50 words.

Another factor that may influence children's use of new words is unsolicited imitation. Although young children vary considerably in the degree to which they engage in such behavior, imitation seems to play a role in lexical acquisition for those children who do imitate. Two hypotheses concerning the influence of imitation on lexical acquisition have been explored. The first is that imitated words are acquired more readily in production as a result of the imitation process. This hypothesis is at the heart of studies conducted by Bloom, Hood, and Lightbown (1974) and Ramer (1976). These investigators examined the lexical items used by young children and determined whether such usage was imitative or spontaneous. They found it was proper to speak of two populations of words in a child's speech—words used spontaneously and words used imitatively. Further, they observed a progression across time as imitation of a particular lexical item decreased while the spontaneous use of the lexical item increased. Such findings led to the interpretation that imitation could serve as a vehicle through which words might be introduced more readily into the lexicon. As imitation was not viewed as necessary for the normal acquisition of all of the child's words, the facilitative effects of imitation were assumed to apply only to those words the child chose to imitate.

More recently, a second hypothesis has been investigated. Leonard, Schwartz, Folger, Newhoff, and Wilcox (1979) attempted to determine whether imitated words were acquired more readily in production than words that were not imitated. These investigators presented novel words and their referents to children in sessions designed to simulate informal play. During these sessions, the children's imitative and spontaneous use of the words was noted. Leonard et al. observed that the first spontaneous use of nonimitated words required no more stimulus exposures than the first spontaneous use of previously imitated words. However, in a follow-up study, Leonard, Chapman, Rowan, and Weiss (1983) observed that spontaneous usage was more frequent for words that had been both imitated and used spontaneously (regardless of whether imitation preceded spontaneous use or vice versa) than for words that had been used spontaneously without having been imitated. In addition, words that were produced correctly on a post test were usually those that had been previously imitated. These findings led Leonard et al. to propose that imitation may facilitate lexical acquisition.

Until the mid-1970s, studies of children's early word usage centered principally on the types of words produced (e.g., Nelson, 1973) and the semantic boundaries reflected in such usage (Clark, 1973). In recent years, increasing attention has been placed on the communicative functions served by the child's early word usage (Coggins & Carpenter, 1981; Dale, 1980; Halliday, 1975). One of the most detailed studies on this topic is that of McShane (1980), in which the communicative functions expressed by six children—presented in Table 1-1— were studied longitudinally from approximately age 12 to 24 months. Communicative attempts by the child were assigned to one of the communicative function categories along with a designation of whether the attempt was expressed lexically.

Not surprisingly, the percentage of communicative attempts taking lexical form increased with age. The communicative functions expressed most frequently in lexical form were requests, naming, and answers. However, each of the six children also used lexical items to serve attention, description, information, giving, doing, imitation, follow-on, and question functions. Five of the six children used words to express a determination function. These findings suggest that young children used their relatively limited lexicons to convey a variety of communicative intentions.

The recent findings concerning young children's word productions and the factors influencing them seem to offer some new considerations for clinical management. If language-disordered children are found to show the same phonological selection and avoidance tendencies seen in young normally developing children, it would appear that an additional factor could be considered when selecting the words to include in lexical training. That is, along with selecting words according to their communicative significance for the child (Holland, 1975) and their semantic properties (Lahey & Bloom, 1977), the phonological composition of the words relative to the child's own phonological characteristics might be considered. For example, it could prove useful to select for training those words that conform to the child's phonological characteristics, particularly if a priority is being placed on increasing lexicon size as efficiently as possible.

A finding that unsolicited imitation facilitates the acquisition of words in language-disordered children might also have implications for clinical management. Such a finding could suggest a possible modification in current lexical-training procedures. Specifically, it might prove useful to provide a number of exposures of a word to which the child need not respond (but may choose to imitate) in addition to the formal stimuli (e.g., imitative prompts, questions) to which the child is required to respond.

At present, relatively little is known about the communicative functions served by the early lexical usage of language-disordered children. However, judging from the available data for young normally developing children, there are a variety of communicative uses to which a relatively limited expressive lexicon can be put. It might be important, therefore, to insure that our lexical-training procedures include provisions for associating a new word with more than one communicative function where applicable. Before a child is assumed to have acquired the use of a word, he or she might be required to use it in more than one way (e.g., requesting and naming; doing and description). If a child has acquired the use of a number of words, yet fails to use any to serve a particular communicative function typically seen in young normally developing children, specific attempts to increase awareness of this function might be instituted.

Language Learning Styles

In recent years, one of the most important lessons we have learned about young children's language development is that children may follow different routes, yet still acquire language in a normal manner and at a normal rate. The study that first opened our eyes to this fact was performed by Nelson (1973). In an examination of the first 50 words used by young normally developing children, Nelson observed some clear differences in the distribution of words across lexical categories. The most striking differences between the children was in the number of general nominals used, such as names of objects, animals, and substances. Over half of the lexical items used by some of the children took the form of general nominals. These children were termed "referential speakers" since they seemed to display an object-oriented language. The other children—termed "expressive speakers"—made less use of general nominals and appeared to display a social-interaction language. Compared to the referential speakers, the expressive speakers showed greater use of personal-social words, such as *pat-a-cake* and *whoops*. These differences in lexical orientation were related to later differences between the children. For example, at 24 months of age, the referential speakers displayed larger vocabularies than the expressive speakers (see, also, Nelson, 1975). On the other hand, the expressive speakers used a larger number of phrases early in the language-acquisition period than did the referential speakers. The latter group appeared, instead, to follow a gradual progression from the single- to the two-word-utterance stage.

It now seems that the styles identified by Nelson (1973) may apply as well to young children who have been studied by other investigators. For example, Dore (1974) observed the linguistic development of two children and noted that one child used many object names and progressed from the single- to the two-word stage in a discrete fashion, while the other child, from the outset, used a number of phrases identifiable more from their intonation than from their phonetic accuracy. Peters (1977) also described a young child with limited intelligibility who used phrases identifiable from their intonation contours, as well as a number of personal-social words. Other investigators have observed differences in lexical usage

Table 1-1
McShane's (1980) Communicative function categories.

CATEGORY	DEFINITION	EXAMPLE
Regulation		
Attention	An utterance that attempts to direct the attention of another person to an object or event.	.*look,* as the child points to an object and looks up at the listener.
Request	An utterance that requests that another person do something for the child, or requests permission to do something.	*juice,* as the child holds out a glass to the mother.
Vocative	An utterance that calls another person to locate him or her or to request his or her presence.	*Mommy* (spoken loudly) as the child goes from room to room in search of mother.
Statement		
Naming	An utterance that makes reference to an object or person by name only.	*car,* as the child points to a car.
Description	An utterance that makes some statement, other than naming, about an object, action, or event.	*gone,* as the child arrives at the location where a desired object is usually found, but is unable to find it.

Table 1-1
McShane's (1980) Communicative function categories.

CATEGORY	DEFINITION	EXAMPLE
Information	An utterance that makes a statement about an event beyond the "here-and-now;"excluding acts the child is about to perform.	*chick*, as the child looks at the visitor. The mother then comments "We saw some chicks at the farm yesterday, didn't we?"
Exchange		
Giving	An utterance spoken while giving or attempting to give an object to another person.	*here*, as the child hands a doll to the father.
Receiving	An utterance spoken while receiving an object from another person.	*thank you*, as the child takes the offered cookie.
Personal		
Doing	An utterance describing an act the child is performing or has just performed.	*down*, after the child has just put a box of blocks on the floor.
Determination	An utterance specifying the child's intention to carry out some act immediately.	*out*, spoken immediately before standing up and walking toward the door.

Table 1-1
McShane's (1980) Communicative function categories.

CATEGORY	DEFINITION	EXAMPLE
Refusal	An utterance used to refuse an object or request to do something.	*no*, as the mother hands the child a hat to put on the doll.
Protest	A "high-pitched" utterance expressing the child's displeasure with an action by another person.	*don't!*, as the child's brother starts to take the play phone away from the child.
Conversation *Imitation*	An utterance that imitates all or part of a preceding adult utterance with no intervening utterance on the child's part.	*fish*, in response to the father's utterance "What a big fish."
Answer	An utterance spoken in response to a question (excluding imitations).	*shoe*, in response to the mother's question "What's this called?"
Follow-on	An utterance serving as a conversational response that is neither an imitation nor an answer.	*yeah*, in response to the visitor's comment "Let's see what's in the box."
Question	An utterance that requests information from another person.	*what's that?*, as the child looks first at a microphone, then at the visitor.

(Snyder, Bates, & Bretherton, 1979), the types of multi-word utterances acquired (Lieven, 1980) and patterns of play behavior (Rosenblatt, 1975; Wolf & Gardner, 1979) that may parallel the style differences reported by Nelson. Some caution should be taken in interpreting the literature on language-learning style, however. Nelson (1981) has raised the possibility that the two styles may represent two extremes on a continuum, and that some children may fall at neither extreme. Further, Peters has noted that the speaking situation at hand may dictate the degree to which a child exhibits behaviors associated with one or another style.

Assuming that style distinctions can be made with language-disordered children, determination of a child's style may have important implications for the selection of additional words to include in lexical training. A study of young normally developing children by Leonard et al. (1981) offers an illustration. These investigators presented novel object and action words and referents to referential and expressive speakers for 10 sessions. The referential speakers acquired a greater number of the object words than the expressive speakers. However, the two groups did not differ in their acquisition of the action words. Such a finding suggests that for language-disordered children exhibiting a referential style, introduction of new general nominals might lead to more rapid lexical learning than would be the case if other types of words had been selected for training. At some point, of course, such a concentration on words of a particular type should give way to a more balanced distribution of lexical types. However, this approach of selecting words in keeping with a child's language-learning style may have some benefits in cases where the child's lexical growth is proceeding rather slowly.

Early Combinatorial Speech

Early Comprehension of Word Combinations
Prior to their production of true word combinations, young children show evidence of comprehending two-word utterances to a limited degree. In some cases this comprehension may be more apparent than real, as when a child responds correctly to the request "Throw ball," not because he or she understood the relational aspects of the utterance, but because he or she understood the word "ball" and performed the action typically associated with the ball (Chapman, 1978). However, there is evidence that children at this stage in linguistic development can make inferences about the relationship between two words. Sachs and Truswell (1978) presented young children with a comprehension task involving familiar words in novel combinations arranged in sets of four-way minimal contrasts (e.g., "Pat

teddy, " "Kiss book, " "Pat book, " "Kiss teddy"). Ten of the 12 children studied performed well on this task and the remaining children responded correctly to some of the instructions. It should be noted that this did not constitute evidence of syntatic comprehension, for the children's responses to requests such as "Teddy kiss" were not tested. It is possible that under such circumstances children might adopt the strategy of acting as agent themselves (Chapman, 1978). However, their successful performance on the Sachs and Truswell task indicates that late in the single-word utterance stage, children can process more than one word in the utterances directed toward them.

The Sachs and Truswell (1978) task seems to have considerable potential for use in clinical settings. Through use of minimal contrasts, non-linguistic and single-lexical-item response strategies are obviated, enabling the clinician to determine whether the child can comprehend both components of certain two-word utterances. Successful performance on this task might serve as a criterion for the child's entry into two-word-utterance production training.

Two Word Utterance Usage

For more than a decade, the study of children's two-word utterances has included a consideration of the types of meanings they convey. This work has led to the impression that, regardless of the language being acquired, young children seem to express the same relatively small set of meanings. These include noting identification, disappearance, recurrence, location, or properties of things, as well as the actions of those things, and the agents performing these actions.

In the past few years, however, the analysis of the relational meanings reflected in children's early word combinations has seemed much less straightforward than previously presumed. During this period, several papers have pointed out a number of difficulties involved in placing two-word utterances into semantic-relation categories (Duchan & Lund, 1979; Howe, 1976; 1981; Rodgon, 1977). The most serious problem is that the semantic relations often ascribed to children may not reflect the relational meanings that are actually operative in their speech. This concern has been tempered somewhat by recent arguments that the analysis of children's utterances in their situational context does not constitute imposing adult semantic categories upon the data, but rather deriving categories from the data (Bloom, Capatides, & Tackeff, 1981). Nonetheless, all investigators now seem to agree on the importance of securing firm evidence from the child's speech before assuming that a particular semantic relation is operative in his or her linguistic system.

A method of analysis that seems capable of providing such evidence was developed by Braine (1976), and has since been expanded by Ingram (1979). One of the major features of this approach is that the child's word combinations are assumed to be unanalyzed wholes unless the data can show otherwise. This applies not only to highly routinized forms such as "Thank you" and "What's that?"—but also to forms such as "That ball" and "More juice," which, on first impression, might be assumed to have been generated by means of a rule for combining words. Particular attention is paid to whether or not a word that appears in one combination is also seen in combination with other words (e.g., "Throw ball," "Throw block"). The type of meaning that seems to be reflected in these combinations is then examined. Finally, the child's utterances are examined for word combinations that are unlikely to have been heard in the speech of others (e.g., "That feet").

Application of this analysis procedure to young children's word combinations led Braine (1976) to conclude that semantic relation categories such as action + object, possession, and the like may often be inappropriate for these children. For example, some children exhibit word-combination patterns that seem to be lexically based (e.g., "Open box," "Open door," "Open window"). It seems that such patterns represent cases where the child has focused on a particular word in a particular word position, and has observed the words it combines with in the speech of others. Thus, the utterances produced by the child may not have been generated by a rule for combining words. In other cases, the word combinations seem to reflect a productive rule, as evidenced by the use of clearly novel word combinations (e.g., "Open orange" [=Peel the orange], in addition to "Open box," "Open door"). However, the rule still applies only to specific lexical items (e.g., Open + X). When the child's word-combination rules transcend specific lexical items, they often embody meanings that are too narrow for the traditional semantic-relation categories. For example, Braine has reported evidence for a word-combining rule that might be characterized as Act-of-Oral-Consumption + Object-Consumed (e.g., "Eat banana," "Bite banana," "Eat cookie," "Bite cookie". This is to say that positional consistency obtained only in word combinations related to the acts of eating and drinking.

Thus, these findings indicate that young children's two-word utterances may represent (1) memorization of a number of combinations into which particular words may enter, (2) productive rules applied only to specific words, (3) productive rules conveying meanings that cross lexical boundaries, but are narrower than traditional semantic relation categories, as well as (4) semantic relation rules of the traditional type. Such findings suggest that the assessment of the meanings reflected in the two-word utterances of language-disordered children should be performed with greater care than previously presumed. There seem to be two ways of accomplishing this. One way is to collect speech samples from the child that are larger than the 50- or 100-utterance samples ordinarily obtained in clinical settings. A second approach is to follow up a standard (smaller) speech sample with probes aimed at discovering the bases and nature of the two-word utterances noted in the sample. For example, if the utterance "Little baby" was noted in a child's sample, the clinician might select object and/or pictorial stimuli designed to determine whether the child can use "Little " in combination with other words, whether his or her use of "Little " is part of a relatively narrow word-combining rule (e.g., Size + X, as in "Little baby, " "Little ball, " "Big ball, " "Big dog") or, instead reflects a broader rule that corresponds to a semantic relation such as attribution.

Longer Word Combinations

Shortly after productive two-word utterances are heard in young children's speech, their sentences seem to lengthen almost daily. By the time many children reach two years of age, three-word utterances are almost as common as two-word utterances, and four- and five-word utterances are not out of the ordinary. However, the rapidity of this progression from two-word utterances to those of longer length should not be taken to mean that the process is unpatterned. For example, Bloom, Miller, and Hood (1975) have noted several conditions that seem to increase or decrease the likelihood that an utterance will contain three versus two constituents. While use of verb inflections, prepositions, noun inflections, and determiners seem equally likely in two- or three-constituent utterances, the expression of negation, recurrence, possession, and attribution seem less likely in three-constituent utterances. Similarly, verbs previously used by the child appear as likely to occur in three- as in two-constituent utterances, but newly acquired verbs are usually restricted to two-constituent utterances. Finally, differences can be seen in the distribution of two- and three-constituent utterances in discourse. While two-constituent utterances often serve as the first utterance in a sequence, utterances containing three constituents often serve as expansions of a prior utterance.

The findings of Bloom et al. (1975) seem to have a great deal of potential for clinical application. For example, for language-intervention procedures in which several linguistic features serve as simultaneous goals, the clinician might be able to model certain combinations of features (e.g., Agent + Action + Location utterances which also contain a preposition such as "Mommy sit on bed") that, when attempted by the child, have a reasonable likelihood of being produced accurately. If children prove more able to produce three-constituent utterances when such utterances serve as expansions, the clinician employing a modeling approach might alter the procedure to accommodate such expansions. For example, rather than describing three pictures using an Agent + Action + Object construction and then presenting the child with a fourth picture to which he or she is asked to respond, the clinician might describe each of the three pictures with a two-part response, composed of a two-constituent description followed by a three-constituent expansion (e.g., "Ride bike." "Daddy ride bike."). The clinician might then provide a two-constituent description of a fourth picture and ask the child to provide the follow-up utterance. Finally, the Bloom et al. findings regarding the relative use of new and old lexical items in three-constituent utterances suggest that training activities designed to facilitate the child's production of longer utterances should make use of lexical items, particularly action words, which the child has been using for some time (Bloom & Lahey, 1978).

Grammatical Inflections

As children's utterances increase in length, function words and grammatical inflections begin to appear. Fourteen of these words and inflections comprise the grammatical morphemes examined in Brown's (1973) well-known longitudinal study. He noted that these morphemes are acquired in an approximately consistent order across children, a finding generally supported by the cross-sectional findings of deVilliers and deVilliers (1973). While Brown found evidence that the syntactic and/or semantic complexity of the morphemes may be partly responsible for their order of acquisition, he found no evidence that acquisition order was related to the frequency with which the morphemes were used in parental speech. More recently, a lively debate has surfaced in which it has been claimed, after further analysis of Brown's data, that parental input frequency is a factor in acquisition order (Moerk, 1980) and that syntactic and semantic complexity are not (Block & Kessel, 1980). Pinker (1981) has re-examined each of these newer claims in detail and has concluded that they are based on faulty interpretations of the statistical analysis used. Pinker's arguments appear reasonable and, thus, for the time being, Brown's original conclusions still stand.

Investigations of children's use of grammatical inflections have not been limited to those concerned with the sequence in which inflections appear, or the factors responsible for this sequence. One of the most informative studies pertaining to grammatical inflections, in fact, dealt with the types of verbs with which the verb inflections -*ing,* -*s* and -*ed* (the latter considered along with irregular past forms) typically co-occur in young children's speech (Bloom, Lifter, & Hafitz, 1980). Action verbs that occurred with -*ing* were found to name events extending over time (durative) in which there was no immediate and clear result (noncompletive). Examples include *play, ride,* and *write.* The action verbs associated with -*s* were typically completive and durative, in that the completed action leaves a relatively permanent state of affairs, as seen in "This goes here" or "It fits." Action verbs associated with -*ed* and irregular usage usually named nondurative, completive events (e.g., *jump, bite*). The tendency for an action verb to be associated primarily with one type of inflection was seen principally when the verb was newly acquired. Unlike most action verbs, those that seemed to serve as "all-purpose" verbs with rather general meanings (e.g., *do, make, get*) often occurred with more than one inflection.

Bloom et al. (1980) also noted a difference between types of state verbs. Those that named internal, nonshared events, such as *want* and *like,* were rarely inflected. However, those that referred to observable processes (e.g., *look, lay, sleep*) were more likely to be inflected.

The finding that young children seemed to make use of different inflections according to whether a verb is durative or nondurative, or completive or noncompletive, led Bloom et al. (1980) to propose that aspect rather than tense may motivate children's early inflectional usage. That is, the use of verb inflections did not seem closely tied to the relationship between the time that the action or state occurred and the time when the utterance referring to the action or state was produced. This usage did seem related to the temporal contour of particular events, however, such as whether an action was momentary in time or extended over a considerable period of time.

The Bloom et al. (1980) findings make it clear that when teaching language-disordered children the use of verb inflections, considerable attention should be paid to the semantics of the verbs used. It seems more likely that the durative, noncompletive nature of verbs such as *play* may be particularly conducive to -*ing* training, while the nondurative, completive character of verbs such as *jump* may facilitate the acquisition of -*ed.* The use of -*s* might be fostered by the introduction of completive, but durative, verbs such as *fit.* At some point, of course, the child will need to demonstrate evidence of the ability to use more than one inflection with the same verb. Training activities with this as their goal might include in the early stages "all-purpose" verbs (e.g., *do, make*) whose meanings are sufficiently broad to accommodate a number of aspectual contours.

Conversational Skills

Contingent and Adjacent Speech

The child-language literature since the mid-1970s has reflected a growing interest in the nature of the development of children's conversational skills. One area of investigation has been the relationship between the child's utterances and preceding adult utterances, and how this relationship changes across time. The available evidence suggests that from at least the age of 21 months, children's utterances more often than not temporally follow an adult utterance (Bloom, Rocissano, & Hood, 1976). However, approximately one-third of these adjacent utterances do not share the same topic as the prior adult utterance. Another 10% to 25% represent imitations of the adult utterance. Contingent utterances—those that share the same topic and add new information—represent approximately 25% of the child's adjacent utterances. Bloom et al. noted that by the time the child has reached three years of age, the percentage of adjacent utterances falling into the first two categories is much lower, while contingent speech may represent as much as 50% of the child's adjacent speech.

The fact that children's unsolicited imitations are quite frequent at a point in their development when their contingent speech is low has led a number of investigators to propose that one function of imitation may be to enable children to participate in conversation at a time when their limited linguistic ability restricts the amount of original and relevant information they can provide (Keenan, 1974; Mayer & Valian, 1977; McTear, 1978). Only Boskey and Nelson (1980) have studied this issue in systematic fashion, by asking children predesigned questions that they could and could not answer during the course of a play activity. Boskey and Nelson found unanswerable questions were likely to result in imitation, while relevant verbal responses were more frequent for answerable questions. Thus, some support can be found for the hypothesis that young children may imitate when they have nothing else to say. Along with facilitating the child's acquisition of specific linguistic materal (as discussed above), then, imitation may assist the child during conversational participation.

It appears that children's developing use of contingent speech represents more than a simple increase in the proportion of adjacent utterances that add new information to the topic. Bloom et al. (1976) noted that the proportion of contingent utterances that followed from the situation or action pertaining to the adult's utterance (contextually contingent speech) decreased across time, while the proportion of contingent utterances showing structural continuities with the clause structure of the adult utterance (linguistically contingent speech) increased. Two main types of linguistically contingent speech were identified. The first type involved intraclausal relations, in which the child's utterance changed or added information to the same clause structure seen in the adult utterance. Interclausal relations represented the second type. In this case, the child's utterance added information with another clause that was grammatically subordinate to the clause of the adult utterance. Both types of linguistically contingent speech increased across time relative to the use of contextually contingent speech. However, utterances involving interclausal relations emerged several months after those involving intraclausal relations.

One form of contingent speech that has received considerable investigative attention is the contingent query, a device seemingly used by the child to regulate the verbal interaction. Research conducted by Garvey (1977; 1979) indicates that the various forms of the contingent query are well learned by three years of age. Contingent queries seem to serve several different functions. They can serve as requests for repetition, confirmation, specification, or elaboration. Examples of each of these functions appear in Table 1-2.

An inspection of the types of utterances young children use following an utterance by their co-conversationalist offers a number of insights regarding possible intervention strategies with language-disordered children. First, it appears that the child's use of imitation during conversation might be regarded as an acceptable response to a preceding utterance by another. As there is no evidence to date that imitation facilitates the child's acquisition of new conversational devices, it should probably not represent a target for training. However, the information contained in the child's imitation could be acknowledged and the imitation itself accepted as an appropriate conversational turn, unless the clinician has reason to believe the child can respond with an information-bearing comment of his or her own.

Active attempts to teach the child the use of contingent speech might commence with intraclausal relations between the adult utterance and the child's response. For example, within a modeling framework, the clinician might present a picture to the model and child, saying "The truck is pulling a car." The model might respond with "A broken car" or "Train can pull car. " Providing the child with a number of such examples might enable him or her to discover some ways to add information to a preceding utterance produced by another. Once a child shows use of contingent speech involving intraclausal relations, modeling might focus on interclausal relations. Contingent utterances of this type seem to require greater grammatical sophistication on the child's part. Therefore, it would be necessary to precede such training with a careful consideration of the child's grammatical skills. Examples of interclausal relations might include the clinician's description of a picture, "The girl is carrying some popcorn," followed by the model's comment "She's gonna eat it."

Table 1-2
Illustration of the functions of contingent queries proposed by Garvey (1979).

FUNCTION	PRECEDING UTTERANCE	CONTINGENT QUERY*
Request for Repetition	"Let's take the truck."	"The what ∕"
Request for Confirmation	"The bike is too small for Daddy."	"The black one ∕"
Request for Specification	"Hold onto the box. You don't want to break it."	"What ∖"
Request for Elaboration	"Hurry up. We're gonna go now."	"Where ∖"

*∕ indicates phrase-final rise in intonation, ∖ indicates phrase-final fall in intonation.

The specific functions served by contingent queries make them good candidates for inclusion in a language-treatment program. Contingent queries serve as signals to the co-conversationalist that the message was not fully understood. The specific form of the query indicates to the co-conversationalist which aspect of the message needs to be repeated, specified, etc. Given that a number of language-disordered children experience comprehension difficulties, a means to indicate that a message was not fully understood as spoken would be highly useful. Again, a modeling framework might be appropriate. For example, the clinician might tell a brief story about two girls who are bored and who decide they are going to go outside "to look for it" (deliberately not being clear as to the referent). The model might then respond, "What ∖," a query for specification. Following a number of queries by the model, the child could be given the charge of providing feedback to the clinician.

Turn-Taking

Another area of active research in recent years is that of children's conversational turn-taking. Much of this work has focused on child-child interactions. Although children seem to be provided with a framework for turn-taking when they are still infants (Ninio & Bruner, 1978), it appears that the proper timing and monitoring of turns are not well established until the early elementary school years. For example, while children six to eight years of age show only minimal overlap in their conversational turns, overlap is much higher in children under four-and-one-half years of age. These younger children are also less able to time their interruptions so they occur at a syntactic or prosodic boundary in the other speaker's utterance. Not surprisingly, younger children show greater difficulty in timing during triadic versus dyadic interaction than older children (Ervin-Tripp, 1979). Along with impressions of the nature and frequency of interruptions, we have impressions of children's reactions to interruptions. Common remedies, regardless of age, seem to be immediate repetition or an increase in volume. Children above the age of four-and-one-half years, however, seem less likely to ignore interruptions than younger children. Frequently, these children stop speaking when such interruptions occur (Ervin-Tripp, 1979).

Of course, not all turn exchanges are mistimed. Garvey and Berninger (1981) have attempted to determine the duration of the pause between one child's utterance and the follow-up utterance of a second child. Such switching pauses are shorter for children approximately five years of age than for children approximately three years of age. For both age groups, pauses are relatively short when the first utterance follows a conventional pattern, has a predictable response, and the response can be selected from a limited set of alternatives or involves only repetition or confirmation:

Child A: "I know where this goes."
Child B: "Where \ "

However, pauses are longer for cases where the response is both less predictable and requires the formulation of linguistic elements new to the discourse:

Child A: "What do you call this?"
Child B: "I'm not sure. Maybe an igloo."

Garvey and Berninger (1981) have also studied the behavior of children when they receive no response to an utterance for which one was expected. In these cases, younger as well as older children seem to follow up their original utterance with another. Repetition appears to be most frequent followed by a change of force (e.g., "I'm going to put this near the window. . .All right?") and paraphrase. Older children seem more likely than younger children to follow up with a change of force if the original utterance was a declarative. Finally, older children seem to wait longer for a response than younger children if the original utterance was an interrogative. Garvey and Berninger suggest that older children may have more confidence in the turn-transfer effects of interrogatives.

The available evidence regarding children's developing turn-taking skills has implications for intervention. For example, children for whom conversational turn-taking is a clinical goal might first be encouraged to participate in dyads. If a child must interact with more than one other child at a time, as is often the case in some preschool language-stimulation programs, the child's conversations may amount to frequent and ill-timed interruptions—or the opposite extreme, a reluctance to actively participate. Triadic communication, then, might be reserved as a later goal of intervention. A child's ability to take conversational turns might be promoted by insuring that a number of the utterances initially directed his or her way have predictable responses whose formulation can be based on a small set of response alternatives, and where, in some cases, simple repetition or confirmation is appropriate.

Wh-Questions

It seems safe to say that one of the reasons why clinicians pay close attention to the literature on normal children's language acquisition is to collect information concerning the sequence in which particular linguistic features might be taught to language-disordered children. In no area is this more true than in the area of *wh*-question acquisition. Previous research with normally developing children has suggested that *wh*-questions emerge in a particular sequence. *What* and *where* questions emerge relatively early, for example, while *why* and *when* questions appear later. These findings have provided clinicians with an approximate order in which *wh*-questions might be trained.

In the past five years, however, we have learned a great deal more about factors that may contribute to the observed sequence of acquisition, and the specific conditions that must be present in order for the sequence to hold. For example, Tyack and Ingram (1977) found that the transitivity of the verb and the sentence constituent represented by the *wh*-word influenced the *wh*-question comprehension of children aged four to five-and-one-half years. While *where* questions containing intransitive verbs were relatively easy for the children, *where* questions with transitive verbs were more difficult. Questions in which *who* served as the object of the sentence ("Who is the girl touching?") were more likely to be comprehended than questions in which *who* served as the subject of the sentence ("Who is touching the girl?").

An investigation by Wootten, Merkin, Hood, and Bloom (1979) has provided considerable insight into the factors involved in the sequence of acquisition seen in children's production of *wh*-questions. The children, studied from approximately 22 to 36 months of age, showed the same general order of acquisition reported in earlier studies, with *what* and *where* questions emerging early, followed by *how, who,* and *why* questions. This sequence seemed attributable in part to the syntactic function served by the *wh*-words. With the exception of *who,* those that serve as *wh*-pronominals asking for the particular constituent they replace, such as *what* or *where,* tended to appear earlier in the children's speech. Those that are *wh*-sententials asking for information pertaining to semantic relations among all the constituents of a sentence (*how* and *why*), appeared later. The somewhat late appearance of *who* questions seemed due to the fact that, unlike the other *wh*-pronominals, *who* was not used by the children in identifying questions (such as "Who's that?") during the early phases of the study. This may have been due to the fact that, at younger ages, children's contact with persons whose identity they might question is relatively limited.

Another factor that Wootten et al. (1979) identified as having a possible bearing on the observed order of emergence was the distribution of verb types with *wh*-words. *What, where,* and *who* questions usually occurred with the copula or the pro-verbs *do* and *go. How* questions were used with verbs that named specific actions and states (*eat, sleep*), as well as with pro-verbs and the copula. *Why* questions, on the other hand, were primarily used with verbs that referred to specific actions and states. This finding suggested the presence of a developmental interaction between the syntactic function of a *wh*-word and the semantic complexity of the verbs used with it.

Finally, Wootten et al. (1979) examined the children's use of *wh*-questions containing no verbs. Those that represented agrammatical constructions ("Where dog?") decreased in frequency over time. On the other hand, an increase across time was seen in the frequency of questions that were elliptical ("What book?" "Why?"), serving as responses to an utterance produced by another.

These recent findings provide additional details that should probably be considered when teaching *wh*-questions to language-disordered children. Although the order of emergence of *wh*-questions reflected in the literature can serve as a general guide for training, it seems essential that the clinician insure that the particular features of *wh*-questions responsible for this order be incorporated into training. For example, *what* questions may be taught first, but only those that serve as identifying questions. Other types of *what* questions might be introduced later. *Where* questions containing intransitive verbs should probably be introduced before those that contain transitive verbs. The acquisition of the later-emerging questions, such as *how* and particularly *why,* seem to be predicated on an ability to use a variety of verbs referring to specific states and actions. Therefore, it would seem important to conduct a detailed assessment of a child's ability with specific verbs before such *wh*-questions are introduced in training.

Complex Sentences

Structure and Meaning

Not long after their second birthday, young children begin to show use of complex sentences that are built up of combinations of simpler sentences. This building-up process can be accomplished through use of one of three different types of syntactic structures. In one type, the simpler sentences are joined by a co-ordinating conjunction such that neither component is subordinate to the other. The second type involves complementation, in which a subordinate sentence fills an empty syntactic slot (e.g., direct object) of the sentence into which it is embedded ("I like eating ice cream"). The third type involves relativization. In this case, a subordinate sentence modifies a constituent of the sentence into which it is embedded (e.g., "There's the man who talks to chairs").

Children's acquisition of complex sentences does not vary only according to the type of syntactic structure involved. Additionally, it varies according to (1) whether or not a sentence connective is used (e.g., *and, because, what, that*), (2) the semantic relations expressed in the complex sentence, and (3) the presence of certain syntactic and/or cognitive processing constraints associated with the complex sentence. For example, when complex sentences containing connectives are considered, it appears that conjunction structures generally emerge in children's speech before structures involving complementation, while complementation structures emerge before structures with relativization (Bloom, Lahey, Hood, Lifter, & Fiess, 1980). However, the first complex sentences in children's speech involve object complementation where no connective is required, as in "I want see Ernie" (Limber, 1973). Sentences of this type often emerge shortly after the same verbs have been used with direct objects, as in "I want car" (Bowerman, 1979). Even conjunction structures first appear as juxtaposed sentences with no connective, such as "(There) my paper, pencil" (Clancey, Jacobsen, & Silva, 1976; Limber, 1973).

An examination of the order of emergence of sentence connectives reveals only a rough order of acquisition, for certain connectives seem quite variable in their point of emergence. The connective *and* typically appears before all others. The connectives *and then* and *because* are usually among the first several to emerge, *that* and *how* among the last (Bloom et al., 1980; Bowerman, 1979). As noted above, this general order may be due in part to the type of syntactic structure in which each connective is involved. For example, *and, and then,* and *because* are often used in conjunction structures, *how* in complementation structures and *that* in complementation and relativization structures.

The sequence of emergence of connectives also seems related to the semantic relations into which they may enter. Bloom et al. (1980) identified a number of such relations in their data. Additive relations were observed quite early. These involved the simple joining of elements whose combination did not create a meaning different from the meaning of each element separately ("Maybe you can carry that and I can carry this"). Other early emerging relations were temporal in character, in which one element of the sentence typically described an event that preceded or followed in time the event noted in the other element, as in "I going this way to get the groceries, then come back." Causal relations, too, emerged relatively early. In sentences of this type, one element of the sentence usually referred to an intended or ongoing action, and the other provided a reason for, or result of, the action ("Get them 'cause I want it"). Among the later emerging relations were adversative and notice relations. The former represented cases in which the information in one element contrasted with that of the other, as in " 'Cause I was tired. But now I'm not tired." Notice relations were seen when the first element of the sentence called attention to a state or action mentioned in the second ("Watch what I'm doing"). Bloom et al. noted that the connective *and* was often used with additive, temporal, and causal relations (among others), *and then* with temporal relations, *because* with causal relations. Later emerging connectives, on the other hand, were more often used with later emerging semantic relations, or were not used frequently with any other semantic relations.

An investigation focusing specifically on causal relations was performed by Hood and Bloom (1979). They noted that children's early expressions of causality make reference to the nonoccurrence of an event or the nonexistence of a state of affairs ("It can't go, 'cause it's too little"), requests for action by the listener ("Move over. Because the train hurt you"), and intended actions ("I want some milk 'cause I have a cold). Bloom and Hood observed differences among their subjects in terms of whether the cause element of the utterance typically preceded or followed the effect element. Interestingly, these order differences seemed to be established before the children began to use connectives. Further, for most of the children, it appears that the dominant order could have dictated which connective was acquired first. Those children who showed a dominant cause/effect order acquired *so* before *because*. Those who exhibited an effect/cause tendency acquired *because* before *so*. The children who showed no preferred order began to use *so* and *because* at approximately the same point in time.

Several studies have reported constraints on the use of certain complex sentences that may relate to processing difficulties and/or the extent to which certain syntactic operations can apply in particular sentence positions. For example, subject complementation and relativization ("The woman who fell went to the hospital") emerge later in children's speech than (nonparticipial) object complementation and relativization, respectively (Limber, 1973). Recently, several studies have focused on the constraints involved in the use of co-ordination with *and*. Lust (1977) presented data from elicited imitation experiments suggesting that young children have difficulty with sentences in which redundant elements have been deleted (phrasal co-ordination, as in, "Mary cooked the meal and ate the bread"), and perform at higher levels with sentences in which redundant elements are included (sentential co-ordination, as in, "Mary cooked the meal and Mary ate the bread"). In addition, when children delete redundant elements, they are more likely to do so when the element to be deleted follows the one to be retained (forward deletion, as in, "Kittens hop and φ run") than when it precedes the element to be retained (backward deletion, as in "Kittens φ and dogs hide").

Unfortunately, the elicited imitation data collected by deVilliers, Tager Flusberg, and Hakuta (1977) were not in accord with those of Lust (1977). These investigators found no evidence that sentential co-ordination was easier than phrasal co-ordination or that forward deletion was more likely than backward deletion. In order to gain greater insight into this issue, deVilliers et al. examined longitudinally collected spontaneous speech samples for instances of co-ordination with *and*. The children were observed to use phrasal co-ordination prior to sentential co-ordination. In addition, cases of forward deletion were more prevalent than those of backward deletion. More recently, Lust and Mervis (1980) performed a cross-sectional examination of young children's spontaneous speech, and reported that cases of forward deletion emerged earlier, and were more frequent, than instances of backward deletion. They also interpreted their data as supporting the view that sentential co-ordination was more frequent in the children's speech than phrasal co-ordination. An examination of their data, however, suggests that this is true only for children at the third highest level of mean-utterance-length studied (mean=4.15 morphemes). Although the evidence reported thus far concerning sentential versus phrasal co-ordination is not sufficiently clear to permit conclusions to be drawn, it does appear that forward deletions are more likely in young children's speech than backward deletions. As noted by deVilliers et al., this may possibly be due to the difficulty of planning for compound sentence subjects, given the right-branching structure of English.

The available evidence regarding children's acquisition of complex sentences offers a number of possibilities for clinical application. It may be important to insure that the child juxtaposes sentences in his or her speech before requiring production of sentences joined by a connective. In the case of causal relations, it might be useful to consider the order in which cause and effect elements are used by the child when selecting the causal connective to introduce in training.

It is clear that the teaching of connectives should involve more than the systematic introduction of connectives in the order seen in normal children's acquisition, with *and* presented before *and then* and *because*, etc. It seems important to insure that an early emerging connective (e.g., *and*) is first trained in utterances that express appropriate early emerging semantic relations (e.g., additive, temporal relations). Whether prior to or after the appearance of sentential conjunction, if it seems helpful to teach a child the use of phrasal conjunction, utterances with forward deletion appear to be the most appropriate to introduce—at least, at the outset.

Finally, the literature suggests that complementation and relativization might be better introduced in object position before subject position during training. It may also prove important to insure that the child can already use complement-taking verbs with direct objects prior to the commencement of complementation training.

Communication Usage

The growing complexity of utterances within the productive capabilities of children approaching age three allows them to use speech in the service of many communicative functions. Dore (1977) has described a number of these functions in a study of the speech used by seven children, ages 34 to 39 months when interacting with their peers and their nursery-school teacher. Thirty-two different functions, or illocutionary acts, were noted in the children's speech. The most common (each constituting from 7% to 10% of the utterances observed) included requests for action, requests for information about the identity, location, or property of an object, labeling of an object or event, descriptions of an event, and reports of the child's internal state. Protests, claims, the expression of rules, compliances with the action requests of others, and requests for permission to perform acts are examples of other functions seen with some regularity. Quite clearly, by the time children reach three years of age their communicative as well as structural capabilities are considerable.

Findings such as Dore's can be valuable to clinicians as guides in selecting communicative situations that might be employed in the clinical setting. It seems reasonable to assume that children who have had practice in using utterances serving a variety of functions may be better able to communicate at home, in the school room, and on the playground. Knowledge of the communicative functions expressed by young children can also provide clinicians with information concerning the lexical and syntactic forms that might be taught to the child. For example, permission requests ("May I go outside?") require the ability to use modals and to transpose elements. The expression of rules ("We should't put our feet on the table") requires use of conditionals and/or modals. Unless the child has acquired these forms, his or her expression of these communicative functions may be quite inadequate.

Texts

Cohesion

Thus far, discussion of children's linguistic development has centered on the comprehension and production of words and sentences. Yet, effective communication often requires the speaker to produce a series of sentences that are logically and structurally connected, as when a story is being told, instructions for the performance of some task are being given, and so on. The process of relating elements of the discourse (or text) together is termed "cohesion." To date, Halliday and Hasan (1976) may have provided the most complete description of the cohesive devices used by competent speakers of the language. These include, among others, anaphoric reference, cataphoric reference, ellipsis, and lexical cohesion. In anaphoric reference, features such as pronouns or definite articles are used to refer back to a previously established referent ("Gina is sick today. She has the flu"). In cataphoric reference, pronouns or demonstratives direct the listener to coming elements of the text ("After he warms up, Edwin is going to be unstoppable"). Ellipsis refers to the deletion of information available in an immediately preceding portion of the text ("Do you like to dance? I do"). In the case of lexical cohesion, a synonym or superordinate is used to refer back to a previously noted referent ("Suddenly, a lion appeared. The beast let out a terrifying roar.").

Relatively little is known about children's use of some of these cohesive devices. It appears that they follow up their own utterances with ellipsis less frequently than those of an interactant, and the percentages of ellipsis of the former type only increase from approximately 10% to 25% during the span from age five through nine years. In addition, for children in this age range, lexical cohesion usually represents no more than repeating the name of a referent in a subsequent utterance, perhaps to signal a continuity of meaning ("Erika wanted to take a walk. But it was raining outside. So Erika watched television instead") (Fine, 1978).

There has been considerable research on both anaphora and cataphora. Much of this work has been concerned with within-sentence anaphoric ("John said that he was going") and cataphoric reference ("Although he was in pain, the runner kept going") (Lust, 1981; Maratsos, 1973; Solan, 1981). However, a few studies focusing on between-sentence anaphora have appeared. These have dealt with use of the definite article. For example, Warden (1976) presented adults and children, ages three, five, seven, and nine years, with three drawings representing sequential events that formed a story. The stories were constructed so that as the subject told a story conforming to the picture sequence, at least two of the referents would each be mentioned twice. Of particular interest to Warden, of course, was whether the children would describe the referent the first time with the indefinite article *a* and, subsequently, with the definite article *the* ("A dog is chasing a hen" [picture 1]. "A cow stops the dog and the hen hides" [picture 2]. "The hen lays an egg" [picture 3]). Warden found that all of the subjects typically used the definite article when describing a referent that had already been mentioned (reaching 100% by age 7). However, the tendency to use the indefinite article when describing a referent introduced for the first time appeared to develop later. Only about one-half of the 3-year-olds' descriptions of newly introduced referents made use of the indefinite article. This percentage was approximately 80% for the 9-year-olds. Using a task similar to that of Warden, Emslie and Stevenson (1981) found evidence that when children are provided with aids to help them remember which referents had and had not appeared before, 3-year-olds' performances more closely approximate that of older children and adults.

Although a great deal more needs to be learned about cohesion in the speech of children, a few features appear in the literature that warrant consideration for possible clinical application. For instance, it seems that ellipsis might be modeled for a child through a two-person interaction in which one speaker's utterance can serve as an elliptical response to an utterance of the other speaker. Given the finding that ellipsis is more likely to follow an utterance of another than an utterance produced by the child, such a tack might be more successful than modeling a monologue in which a speaker responds elliptically to his or her own previous utterance. It also appears that the task used by Warden (1976), and refined by Emslie and Stevenson (1981), serves as an effective means of tapping young children's use of article anaphora, and may therefore prove quite useful as an assessment and/or training procedure with language disordered children.

Story Schemata

A number of psychologists have recently directed their efforts toward a characterization of the structure of stories and other types of prose. This work has indicated that stories, for example, have suprasentential structure, and that persons listening to stories use this structure as an aid to comprehension and recall. The structure of stories has often been described in terms of a grammar consisting of rewrite rules capable of generating well-formed stories, or of breaking them down into constituent units. The constituent units proposed have varied somewhat from investigator to investigator. The story-grammar structure proposed by Mandler and Johnson (1977) involves a setting followed by one or more episodes. Each episode has a beginning, a reaction of a character to the event in the beginning, an attempt to deal with the problem created in the beginning, an outcome of the attempt, and an ending.

When people listen to stories, they use pre-existing schemata acquired through previous experience with the structure of stories, as well as experience with various types of event sequences in the world. These two sources of experience have constituted two interrelated areas of investigation into children's comprehension and recall of stories. Representative of the first area is a study by Mandler (1978). The goal of this study was to determine whether two-episode stories whose structure conformed to the story grammar of Mandler and Johnson (1977) would be better recalled than two-episode stories with a structure characterized by an interleaving of the events of the two episodes. The elementary school-age children serving as subjects recalled more information and showed fewer distortions with the properly structured stories. Interestingly, interleaved stories were often recalled in a properly structured, rather than interleaved, form. Similar findings have been reported by Brown and Murphy (1975) and Stein and Glenn (1979).

As noted above, story schemata that serve as a guide to comprehension and recall are based not only on prior experience with the structure of stories, but also on world knowledge. The latter refers to expectations built up from knowledge of sequences of actions called for in familiar situations. These have been termed "scripts" (Schank & Abelson, 1977). Recently,

McCartney and Nelson (1981) presented evidence that script-based knowledge can play an important role in the story recall of kindergarten and second-grade children. Stories were devised that dealt with activities common to young children, such as eating dinner and preparing for bed. The particular events included in the stories were based, in part, on responses from preschoolers to questions concerning "what happened" during these activities. Along with the events that were hypothesized to conform to the children's scripts, "filler" events were added to the stories. These events enriched the story, but were not central to the activities. McCartney and Nelson found that central events were better recalled than filler events. For example, in a story about dinner time, the children usually recalled the main character being called to dinner, the commencement of eating, and the character's request to be excused, but often failed to recall the announced dinner menu or the topic of conversation during the meal. The older children out-performed the younger children, but primarily in recall of filler events. The two age groups were similar in recalling central events.

It seems that our developing knowledge of the structure of stories might be put to good clinical use. For example, the basic constituents of stories (setting, beginning, reaction, etc.) might be made explicit for language-disordered children, not only to aid comprehension but to serve as a means of ordering their comments when telling a story. The available evidence concerning children's scripts might be used by clinicians as a guide to the kind of information in a story that children may, and may not, be expected to retain. In addition, poor recall of central story events by children who seem to possess sufficient language-comprehension ability for the task might raise the possibility that the child's previous world experience with these events is limited, or is different from that of most children.

Figurative Language

In recent years, a number of studies dealing with children's comprehension and use of nonliteral, or figurative, language have appeared. These investigations have been concerned with riddles, proverbs, idioms, and metaphors. The majority of these studies have focused on metaphors. A metaphor represents the use of words in which one element, the topic, is compared to another, the vehicle, on the basis of shared attributes, the ground (Gardner, Winner, Bechhofer, & Wolf, 1978). For example, in "A shadow is a piece of night, " the topic, "a shadow" is compared to the vehicle, "a piece of night" on the basis of the shared quality of darkness, the ground.

Early work on children's understanding of metaphors suggested that this ability does not appear until children reach approximately nine years of age. However, an abundance of more recent studies suggests that this is not the case. For example, Gardner (1974) found that children as young as 3 years of age could attribute terms such as *happy* and *sad* to colors and auditory tones. Gentner (1977) observed that 4- and 5-year- olds were able to assign body parts (e.g., *knee, mouth*) to pictures of objects such as trees and mountains. These findings suggest that when metaphoric ability is assessed using simple directions, a nonverbal response mode, and familiar words and materials, evidence for metaphoric ability is seen at much younger ages. (In fact, when metaphoric ability is assessed completely independent of language, it is possible that even infants show a limited skill in this area [Wagner, Winner, Cicchetti, & Gardner, 1981]).

Although a basic ability to comprehend metaphoric language emerges early, it is clear that metaphoric ability continues to develop across time. Younger children seem to perform better on metaphors for which they can select the topic that goes with a vehicle provided them (therefore allowing more flexibility in the shared attributes that are criterial) than on metaphors for which all three elements are already provided (Winner, Engel, & Gardner, 1980). They perform better when they can choose from among several possible meanings of a metaphor than when they must explain its meaning (Winner, Rosenthiel, & Gardner, 1976). Not surprisingly, such children understand "frozen" forms, which, due to their frequent use, may have lost their metaphoric quality (e.g., "I ate up a storm") better than novel forms (Pollio & Pollio, 1979). Cross-sensory metaphors ("Her perfume was bright sunshine") are also better understood than psychological-physical metaphors ("The prison guard was a hard rock") (Winner et al., 1976). In addition, similarity metaphors, where objects are compared on the basis of shared features ("The stars are a thousand eyes") seem to be comprehended better by young children than proportional metaphors, where three objects are mentioned and a fourth must be inferred to complete a proportion ("My head is an apple without any core") (Billow, 1975). Performance on each of these more difficult types of metaphors increases with age. Finally, a word should be said about the production of metaphors. Although very young children show evidence of using words that serve as comments of analogy (e.g., Winner, 1979), it is nonetheless the case that the production of novel, appropriate metaphors is infrequent through adolescence, and does not seem to show a developmental increase until after seven years of age (Gardner, Kircher, Winner, & Perkins, 1975).

For many clinicians, a language-disordered child's understanding of metaphoric language would be an achievement beyond expectations.

Indeed, the severity of the linguistic difficulties experienced by many language-disordered children make the acquisition of some of the basic, literal aspects of language enough of a challenge. Nonetheless, figurative language appears not only in conversational speech, but in school activities and upper-elementary-grade textbooks (Ortony, Reynolds, & Arter, 1978). Thus, for the language-disordered child who functions linguistically at or above the four-year level, comprehension of metaphoric ability might constitute a reasonable clinical goal. Much more research needs to be done in this area, but the available work suggests a few directions for possible clinical application. For example, the child might be initially presented with words only, rather than sentences that must be treated in a nonliteral manner. Applying the qualities of the word's referent to referents pertaining to another modality (cross-sensory application) may prove most successful in the early phases of training. Initially, the child might be required only to point to his or her choice. When sentence metaphors are eventually introduced, they might first take the form of similarity metaphors, presented in a multiple-choice-task format.

Summary

In this chapter, a number of findings pertaining to normal language acquisition have been reviewed, with an eye toward how they may have relevance to clinical management. The abilities discussed have ranged from comprehension of the child's first word to appreciation of the relations expressed in a metaphor. The developmental relevance of this literature to clinical activities, then, is difficult to deny. Less certain is the degree to which the reviewed findings should serve as the basis for altering current assessment and training procedures. This question can be answered only if clinicians attempt to incorporate this information in their clinical work, or, better, put some of the possible applications to the test in controlled clinical research.

References

Billow, R. A cognitive developmental study of metaphor comprehension. *Developmental Psychology*, 1975, *11*, 415-423.

Block, E., & Kessel, F. Determinants of the acquisition order of grammatical morphemes: A re-analysis and re-interpretation. *Journal of Child Language*, 1980, *7*, 181-188.

Bloom, L., Capatides, J., & Tackeff, J. Further remarks on interpretive analysis: In response to Christine Howe. *Journal of Child Language*, 1981, *8*, 403-412.

Bloom, L., Hood, L., & Lightbown, P. Imitation in language development: If, when, and why. *Cognitive Psychology*, 1974, *6*, 380-420.

Bloom, L., & Lahey, M. *Language development and language disorders.* New York: Wiley, 1978.

Bloom, L., Lahey, M., Hood, L., Lifter, K., & Fiess, K. Complex sentences: Acquisition of syntactic connectives and the semantic relations they encode. *Journal of Child Language*, 1980, *7*, 235-262.

Bloom, L., Lifter, K., & Hafitz, J. Semantics of verbs and the development of verb inflection in child language. *Language*, 1980, *56*, 386-412.

Bloom, L., Miller, P., & Hood, L. Variation and reduction as aspects of competence in language development. In A. Picke (Ed.), *Minnesota symposia on child psychology* (Vol. 9). Minneapolis: University of Minnesota Press, 1975.

Bloom, L., Rocissano, L., & Hood, L. Adult-child discourse: Developmental interaction between information processing and linguistic knowledge. *Cognitive Psychology*, 1976, *8*, 521-552.

Boskey, M., & Nelson, K. Answering unanswerable questions: The role of imitation. Paper presented to the Boston University Conference on Language Development, Boston, MA., 1980.

Bowerman, M. The acquisition of complex sentences. In P. Fletcher & M. Garman (Eds.), *Language acquisition*. Cambridge, Eng.: Cambridge University Press, 1979.

Braine, M. Children's first word combinations. *Monographs of the Society for Research in Child Development*, 1976, *41* (Serial No. 164).

Brown, A., & Murphy, M. Reconstruction of arbitrary versus logical sequences by preschool children. *Journal of Experimental Child Psychology*, 1975, *20*, 307-326.

Brown, R. *A first language: The early stages*. Cambridge, MA: Harvard University Press, 1973.

Chapman, R. Comprehension strategies in children. In J. Kavanaugh & W. Strange (Eds.), *Speech and language in the laboratory, school, and clinic*. Cambridge, MA: MIT Press, 1978.

Clancey, P., Jacobsen, T., & Silva, M. The acquisition of conjunction: A cross-linguistic study. *Papers and Reports on Child Language Development*, 1976, *12*, 71-80.

Clark, E. What's in a word? On the child's acquisition of semantics in his first language. In T. Moore (Ed.), *Cognitive development and the acquisition of language*. New York: Academic Press, 1973.

Coggins, T., & Carpenter, R. The communicative intention inventory: A system for observing and coding children's early intentional communication. *Applied Psycholinguistics*, 1981, *2*, 235-252.

Dale, P. Is early pragmatic development measurable? *Journal of Child Language*, 1980, *7*, 1-12.

deVilliers, J., & deVilliers, P. A cross-sectional study of the acquisition of grammatical morphemes. *Journal of Psycholinguistic Research*, 1973, *2*, 267-278.

deVilliers, J., Tager Flusberg, H., & Hakuta, K. Deciding among theories of the development of coordination in child speech. *Papers and Reports on Child Language Development*, 1977, *13*, 118-125.

Dore, J. A pragmatic description of early language development. *Journal of Psycholinguistic Research*, 1974, *3*, 343-350.

Dore, J. Children's illocutionary acts. In R. Freedle (Ed.), *Discourse production and comprehension*. Norwood, NJ: Ablex, 1977.

Duchan, J., & Lund, N. Why not semantic relations? *Journal of Child Language*, 1979, *6*, 243-251.

Emslie, H., & Stevenson, R. Pre-school children's use of the articles in definite and indefinite referring expressions. *Journal of Child Language*, 1981, *8*, 313-328.

Ervin-Tripp, S. Children's verbal turn-taking. In E. Ochs & B. Schieffelin (Eds.), *Developmental pragmatics*. New York: Academic Press, 1979.

Ferguson, C., & Farwell, C. Words and sounds in early language acquisition: English initial consonants in the first 50 words. *Language*, 1975, *51*, 419-439.

Ferguson, C., Peizer, D., & Weeks, T. Model and replica phonological grammar of a child's first words. *Lingua*, 1973, *31*, 35-65.

Fine, J. Conversation, cohesive and thematic patterning in children's dialogues. *Discourse Processes*, 1978, *1*, 247-266.

Gardner, H. Metaphors and modalities: How children project polar adjectives onto diverse domains. *Child Development*, 1974, *45*, 84-91.

Gardner, H., Kircher, M., Winner, E., & Perkins, D. Children's metaphoric productions and preferences. *Journal of Child Language*, 1975, *2*, 125-141.

Gardner, H., Winner, E., Bechhofer, R., & Wolf, D. The development of figurative language. In K. Nelson (Ed.), *Children's language* (Vol. 1). New York: Gardner Press, 1978.

Garvey, C. The contingent query: A dependent act in conversation. In M. Lewis & L. Rosenblum (Eds.), *Interaction, conversation, and the development of language*. New York: Wiley, 1977.

Garvey, C. Contingent queries and their relations in discourse. In E. Ochs & B. Schieffelin (Eds.), *Developmental pragmatics*. New York: Academic Press, 1979.

Garvey, C., & Berninger, G. Timing and turn taking in children's conversations. *Discourse Processes*, 1981, *4*, 27-58.

Gentner, D. Children's performance on a spatial analogies task. *Child Development*, 1977, *48*, 1034-1039.

Halliday, M. *Learning how to mean*. London: Edward Arnold, 1975.

Halliday, M., & Hasan, R. *Cohesion in English*. London: Longman, 1976.

Holland, A. Language therapy for children: Some thoughts on context and content. *Journal of Speech and Hearing Disorders*, 1975, *40*, 514-523.

Hood, L., & Bloom, L. What, when, and how about why: A longitudinal study of early expressions of causality. *Monographs of the Society for Research in Child Development*, 1979, *44* (Serial No. 181).

Howe, C. The meanings of two-word utterances in the speech of young children. *Journal of Child Language*, 1976, *3*, 29-47.

Howe, C. Interpretive analysis and role semantics: A ten-year mésalliance? *Journal of Child Language*, 1981, *8*, 439-456.

Huttenlocher, J. The origins of language comprehension. In R. Solso (Ed.), *Theories in cognitive psychology*. Hillsdale, NJ: Lawrence Erlbaum, 1974.

Ingram, D. Early patterns of grammatical development. Paper presented at the Conference on Language Behavior in Infancy and Early Childhood, Santa Barbara, CA, 1979.

Keenan, E. Conversational competence in children. *Journal of Child Language*, 1974, *1*, 163-184.

Lahey, M., & Bloom, L. Planning a first lexicon: Which words to teach first. *Journal of Speech and Hearing Disorders*, 1977, *42*, 340-350.

Leonard, L. Chapman, K., Rowan, L., & Weiss, A. Three hypotheses concerning young children's imitation of lexical items. *Developmental Psychology*, 1983, *19*, 591-601.

Leonard, L., Schwartz, R., Folger, M., Newhoff, M., & Wilcox, M. Children's imitations of lexical items. *Child Development*, 1979, *50*, 19-27.

Leonard, L., Schwartz, R., Morris, B., & Chapman, K. Factors influencing early lexical acquisition: Lexical orientation and phonological composition. *Child Development*, 1981, *52*, 882-887.

Leopold, W. *Speech development of a bilingual child. Volume II. Sound learning in the first two years*. Evanston, IL: Northwestern University Press, 1947.

Lieven, E. Different routes to multiple word combinations? Paper presented at the Stanford Child Language Research Forum, Stanford, 1980.

Limber, J. The genesis of complex sentences. In T. Moore (Ed.), *Cognitive development and the acquisition of language*. New York: Academic Press, 1973.

Lust, B. Conjunction reduction in child language. *Journal of Child Language*, 1977, *4*, 257-288.

Lust, B. Constraints on anaphora in child language: A prediction for a universal. In S. Tavakolian (Ed.), *Language acquisition and linguistic theory*. Cambridge, MA: MIT Press, 1981.

Lust, B., & Mervis, C.A. Development of coordination in the natural speech of young children. *Journal of Child Language*, 1980, *7*, 279-304.

Macken, M. Permitted complexity in phonological development: One child's acquisition of Spanish consonants. *Papers and Reports on Child Language Development*, 1976, *11*, 28-60.

Mandler, J. A code in the node: The use of a story schema in retrieval. *Discourse Processes*, 1978, *1*, 14-35.

Mandler, J., & Johnson, N. Rememberance of things parsed: Story structure and recall. *Cognitive Psychology*, 1977, *9*, 111-151.

Maratsos, M. The effects of stress on the understanding of pronominal coreference in children. *Journal of Psycholinguistic Research*, 1973, *2*, 1-8.

Mayer, J., & Valian, V. When do children imitate? When imitate? When necessary. Paper presented at the Boston University Conference on Language Development, Boston, MA, 1977.

McCartney, K., & Nelson, K. Children's use of scripts in story recall. *Discourse Processes*, 1981, *4*, 59-70.

McShane, J. *Learning to talk*. Cambridge, Eng.: Cambridge University Press, 1980.

McTear, M. Repetition in child language: Imitation or creation? In R. Campbell & P. Smith (Eds.), *Recent advances in the psychology of language: Language development and mother-child interaction*. New York: Plenum Press, 1978.

Menn, L. Phonotactic rules in beginning speech. *Lingua*, 1971, *26*, 225-251.

Menn, L. *Pattern, control, and contrast in beginning speech: A case study in the development of word form and word function*. Unpublished doctoral dissertation, University of Illinois, Champaign, 1976.

Moerk, E. Relationships between parental input frequencies and children's language acquisition: A reanalysis of Brown's data. *Journal of Child Language*, 1980, *7*, 105-118.

Nelson, K. Structure and strategy in learning to talk. *Monographs of the Society for Research in Child Development*, 1973, *38*, Serial No. 1-2.

Nelson, K. The nominal shift in semantic-syntactic development. *Cognitive Psychology*, 1975, *7*, 461-479.

Nelson, K. Individual differences in language development: Implications for development and language. *Developmental Psychology*, 1981, *17*, 170-187.

Ninio, A., & Bruner, J. The achievement and antecedents of labelling. *Journal of Child Language*, 1978, *5*, 1-16.

Ortony, A., Reynolds, R., & Arter, J. Metaphor: Theoretical and empirical research. *Psychological Bulletin*, 1978, *85*, 919-943.

Oviatt, S. The emerging ability to comprehend language: An experimental approach. *Child Development*, 1980, *51* 97-106.

Peters, A. Language learning strategies: Does the whole equal the sum of the parts? *Language*, 1977, *53*, 560-573.

Pinker, S. On the acquisition of grammatical morphemes. *Journal of Child Language*, 1981, *8*, 477-484.

Pollio, M., & Pollio, H. A test of metaphoric comprehension and some preliminary data. *Journal of Child Language*, 1979, *6*, 111-120.

Ramer, A. The function of imitation in child language. *Journal of Speech and Hearing Research*, 1976, *19*, 700-717.

Rodgon, M. Situation and meaning in one- and two-word utterances: Observations on Howe's "The meanings of two word utterances in the speech of young children." *Journal of Child Language*, 1977, *4*, 111-114.

Rosenblatt, D. Learning how to mean: The development of representation in play and language. Paper presented at the Conference on the Biology of Play, Farnham, Eng., 1975.

Sachs, J., & Truswell, L. Comprehension of two-word instructions by children in the one-word stage. *Journal of Child Language*, 1978, *5*, 17-24.

Schank, R., & Abelson, R. *Scripts, plans, goals and understanding.* Hillsdale, NJ: Lawrence Erlbaum, 1977.

Schwartz, R., & Leonard, L. Do children pick and choose? Phonological selection and avoidance in early lexical acquisition. *Journal of Child Language*, 1982, *9*, 319-336.

Shibamoto, J., & Olmsted, D. Lexical and syllabic patterns in phonological acquisition. *Journal of Child Language*, 1978, *5*, 417-456.

Snyder, L., Bates, L., & Bretherton, I. The transition from first words into syntax: Continuities from 13 to 20 months. Paper presented at the Boston University Conference on Language Development, Boston, 1979.

Solan, L. The acquisition of structural restrictions on anaphora. In S. Tavakolian (Ed.), *Language acquisition and linguistic theory.* Cambridge, MA: MIT Press, 1981.

Stein, N., & Glenn, C. An analysis of story comprehension in elementary school children. In R. Freedle (Ed.), *New directions in discourse processing.* Norwood, NJ: Ablex, 1979.

Tyack, D., & Ingram, D. Children's production and comprehension of questions. *Journal of Child Language*, 1977, *4*, 211-224.

Vihman, M. From pre-speech to speech: On early phonology. *Papers and Reports on Child Language Development*, 1976, *12*, 230-244.

Wagner, S., Winner, E., Cicchetti, D., & Gardner, H. "Metaphorical" mapping in human infants. *Child Development*, 1981, *52*, 728-731.

Warden, D. The influence of context on children's use of identifying expressions and references. *British Journal of Psychology*, 1976, *67*, 101-112.

Winner, E. New names for old things: The emergence of metaphoric language. *Journal of Child Language*, 1979, *6*, 469-491.

Winner, E., Engel, M., & Gardner, H. Misunderstanding metaphor: What's the problem? *Journal of Experimental Child Psychology*, 1980, *30*, 22-32.

Winner, E., Rosenthiel, A., & Gardner, H. The development of metaphoric understanding. *Developmental Psychology*, 1976, *12*, 289-297.

Wolf, D., & Gardner, H. Style and sequence in early symbolic play. In N. Smith & M. Franklin (Eds.), *Symbolic functioning in children.* Hillsdale, NJ: Lawrence Erlbaum, 1979.

Wootten, J., Merkin, S., Hood, L., & Bloom, L. *Wh*-questions: Linguistic evidence to explain the sequence of acquisition. Paper presented to the Society for Research in Child Development, San Francisco, 1979.

Jacqueline Weis Liebergott
Anthony S. Bashir
Martin C. Schultz

Dancing Around and Making Strange Noises: Children at Risk

One of the more familiar vaudeville routines goes something like this: "Daddy, why are you out in the backyard dancing around and making strange noises?" "I'm performing an incantation to ward off white elephants," answers the father. Delighted to be able to outwit her father, the child says, "But, Daddy, I don't see any white elephants." And the ever-wise father retorts, "Exactly."

In an attempt to modify, if not ward off, the effects of handicapping conditions, speech-language clinicians are joining with other developmental specialists in early intervention programs for young handicapped and at-risk children. Our involvement in these programs suggests that we share with our colleagues the belief, or hope, that early intervention will enhance the child's developmental status. We also believe that as language clinicians we have a major role in achieving this improved outcome. Inherent in our belief is the idea that we can identify and assess infants and young children who may be at risk for language disorders. Similarly, we believe that we can use our findings to design effective models of intervention, as well as to determine therapeutic goals.

This chapter addresses some of the issues involved in the identification and assessment of children at risk for language impairments. It is apparent that the potential for future developments in these areas will be more exciting than the present state of the art.

© College-Hill Press, Inc. All rights, including that of translation, reserved. No part of this publication may be reproduced without the written permission of the publisher.

At-Risk Children: Problems in Determination

A series of problems and questions arise when the label "at risk" is used to designate the developmental status of a child. The clinician might ask: "What is the child at risk for? What event or criteria did you use in making your determination? What were the key elements in the child's history or the family history that made you concerned for the possibility of later developmental or communicative problems? What clinical assessment scales or measurements were used to determine the child's status?" In answering these questions, different aspects and perspectives concerning the problem emerge. As speech-language clinicians, our primary concern is the identification of those children who are specifically at risk for language problems. As yet, however, we are not able to specify what types of differences in communicative behaviors place the very young child at risk. Consequently, we have relied on approaches that use the presence of a variety of antecedent conditions to say that a child is at risk for future language problems.

Such an approach is seen in the works of Tjossem (1976) and Ramey, Trohanis, and Hostler (1982). They distinguish three kinds of risk factors. These factors are established risk, environmental risk, and biological risk. The groupings are not mutually exclusive.

1. *Established Risk.* "This term refers to the infant whose early appearing and aberrant development is related to diagnosed medical disorders of known etiology and which have relatively well known expectancies for developmental outcome within specified ranges of developmental delay" (Ramey, Trohanis, & Hostler, 1982, p. 8). Children with Down's syndrome, deafness, or hearing impairment are in this category.

2. *Environmental Risk.* "When the life experiences of a biologically sound infant are limited to the extent that, without corrective intervention, they impart a high probability for delayed development, the infant is at environmental risk" (Ramey et al., 1982, p. 8). Notice the tautology implicit in this definition, since the judgment concerning the need for intervention has become part of the definition. Abused and/or neglected children and failure-to-thrive children are suspected by some to be at-risk for a language impairment.

3. *Biological Risk.* "This term specifies the infant who presents a history of prenatal, perinatal, neonatal and early development events suggestive of biological insult to the developing central nervous system and which, either sing-

ly or collectively, increase the probability of later appearing aberrant development" (Ramey et al., 1982, p. 8). Among these conditions are anoxia, very low birth weight, prematurity at birth, respiratory-distress syndrome, metabolic disturbances, and central-nervous-system disorders.

The approach that uses antecedent conditions to identify children at high risk has several inherent problems. First, as pointed out by Cairns and Butterfield (1981), two types of inappropriate expectancies occur. Some of the children with a history of certain antecedent conditions do not develop poorly, while some children with no early indications of problems do not do well. Further, the various categories defining risk represent a not well-understood continuum, and there is uncertainty concerning the eventual communicative status of children in many of these categories. For example, we have more informatioin about the consequences of deafness and Down's syndrome on communicative status than we have about the effects of such conditions as failure to thrive, prematurity of birth, or metabolic disease. Finally, given the variability in outcomes associated with histories of different antecedent conditions, little is to be gained from a *strict* reliance on established, environmental, and biological risk factors for identifying children with potential problems.

To elaborate some of the issues and limitations related to the use of antecedent conditions for determining whether a child is at risk for later language disorders, we have chosen to focus on biological risk factors, specifically infants born prematurely. We first discuss what is known about the existence of handicapping conditions in general in this population, and then describe what is known about their speech and language status.

Prematurity

Field (1979) makes a distinction between "healthy" and "sick" premature infants. "Sick" premature infants are those suffering from complications in addition to prematurity. These complications include asphyxia, respiratory-distress syndrome, metabolic disorders, and such central-nervous-system complications as subependymal-intraventricular hemorrhage. The outcome for infants with one or more of these complications is less favorable than for those who are free of complications.

Approximately 7% of all pregnancies end before term (Pilliteri, 1981). According to Fitzhardinge (1980), in the absence of asphyxia, the prognosis for infants weighing between 1,500 and 2,500 grams is very good. The introduction of the neonatal intensive-care unit and advances in the medical management of these infants have reduced neonatal mortality and morbidity (Field, 1979; Thompson & Reynolds, 1977). For infants weighing between 1,000 and 1,500 grams, survival rates from 1947 to 1968 were 40% to 50%, whereas data collected in the late 1970s showed survival rates approaching 75% to 95% for low-birth-weight infants managed within intensive-care units (ICUs) (Thompson & Reynolds, 1977). Iatrogenic problems of the ICUs of the late 1960s and early 1970s have also decreased, as neonatologists have learned more about appropriate management of respiratory complications, temperature control, and metabolic, biochemical, and nutritional needs (Koops & Harmon, 1980). The outlook for babies born weighing less than 1,000 grams, whose weight is appropriate for their gestational age, is also improving, but Thompson and Reynolds (1977) report that the number of survivors remains below 30%. Similarly, the incidence of severely handicapping conditions in this group remains high. In data reported by Kitchen, Ryan, Rickards, et at., (1980), there was a survival rate of 47.7% for those weighing under 1,000 grams in 1978, as compared to 6.4% in the early 1970s. Changes in numbers of children with serious handicaps have also occurred. For example, Lubchenco (1976), describing children born in the 1950s and early 1960s, reported an incidence of cerebral palsy in low-birth-weight infants of 32%; more recent studies report incidences of cerebral palsy as ranging from 2.4% (Kitchen et al., 1980) to 4% (Fitzhardinge & Ramsay 1973; Stewart & Reynolds, 1974).

Although the presence of severe handicapping conditions has decreased, the numbers of children who have mild and moderate disabilities that may relate to problematic educational outcomes or disruption in social interaction patterns persist. Thompson and Reynolds (1977) state that additional information on the subtle educational, speech, hearing, and behavioral disabilities of low-birth-weight infants is necessary if we are to appreciate the problems encountered by those who survive. Fitzhardinge (1980) suggested that the identification of later language and learning problems evidenced by surviving infants was complicated by the lack of sensitive assessment measures of the less severe conditions.

Studies of speech and language acquisition involving direct assessment of young children's communicative behavior are few. The children evaluated in these studies are sometimes not clearly described and, because evaluation procedures and ages of assessment differ markedly, it is difficult to make comparisons across studies. Furthermore, it is all too obvious that there are insufficient valid and reliable instruments for measuring the language of very young children. This issue is discussed at length in a later section of this chapter.

Kastein and Fowler (1959) reported data on the speech and language abilities of 66 premature infants evaluated at two years of age. No descriptions of what characterized the children's prematurity or their neonatal course were provided. Of these 66 children born at a time when 50% was the survival rate for premature infants, 58% were considered to have "retardations of language and speech development." DeHirsch, Jansky, and Langford (1964) also studied the language abilities of premature children born in the 1950s. They evaluated 51 prematurely born children and 66 maturely born children. The two groups were evaluated at 5.8 years on the average. The premature children had birth weights ranging from 1,000 to 2,239 grams. Both groups had normal intellectual achievement on the Stanford-Binet Intelligence Scale, Form L. Fifteen different measures of speech and language were used. Significant differences were found between the two groups on 7 of the measures: handtapping patterns, language comprehension, word finding, number of words used, mean length of the five longest utterances, sentence elaboration, and definitions. DeHirsch et al. suggested that these differences resulted from the premature children's "lingering neurophysiological immaturity," directing the argument to the issue of delay-versus-deficient language. Unfortunately, the important question—"will the noted language difference affect the child's achievement of educational and social success?—was left unanswered, and remains so to this day.

The results of the Collaborative Perinatal Project of the National Institute of Neurological and Communication Disorders and Stroke (Lassman, Fisch, Vetter, & LaBenz, 1980) provide us with data collected on the largest published sample of premature children evaluated for speech and language abilities. Their sample of approximately 20,000 children included 917 premature children ($\leq$ 36 weeks and $\leq$ 2,500 grams) and 100 low-birth-weight children ($\leq$ 1,500 grams) born in the early 1960s. The speech and language abilities of these children were assessed at 3 and 8 years of age. When the 917 premature children were compared to the entire 8-year-old sample, the premature children performed more poorly in articulation, language comprehension and production, word identification, and concept development. Further, the 100 low-birth-weight children performed even more poorly than the children with birth-weights between 1,500 and 2,500 grams. No tests of statistical significance were performed on these data, since the study designers believed that statistical significance did not necessarily indicate clinical significance. The authors interpreted their findings much like DeHirsch et al., suggesting that eventually the majority of premature children would reach normal developmental levels. Like many others, this study did not address the question of whether or how early reductions in speech and language abilities of these children might be related to later educational status and social development.

Ehrlich, Shapiro, Kimball, and Huttner (1973) evaluated the language and speech abilities of 181 high-risk children at five years of age. Twenty-nine measures were used to assess these children, including the Peabody Picture Vocabulary Test, Templin-Darley Articulation Screening Test, the Illinois Test of Psycholinguistic Abilities, the Wechsler Pre-School and Primary Scale of Intelligence, and the Leiter. Although children having evident neurological abnormalities (reported in their intensive care unit records) were excluded from the study, at the time of the assessment six of the children demonstrated neurologic and sensory problems, three evidenced mild retardation, two had cerebral palsy, two had visual impairments, and two had sensorineural hearing loss. Significant correlations were found between language ability and each of these antecedent conditions: respiratory-distress syndrome, birth weights of less than 2,500 grams, and shortened gestational age. Only 16% of the total sample was functioning normally, 30% was reported as needing "close watching," and 54% was recommended for follow-up.

It is important to remember that the children included in the above reported studies were born in the 1950s and 1960s, a time when catastrophic outcomes were common. What of the children of the 1970s? Fitzhardinge (1980) in a study of full-term, small-for-gestational-age children, reported that 13 of 39 boys and 15 of 67 girls had significant speech problems. Twenty-two children had problems that persisted into school age. She concluded that although improved nutrition during the neonatal period may have reduced the incidence of speech and language delay and disorders below that seen in the survivors of the 1960s, specific learning disabilities and language disorders will most likely be evident in the apparently normal 1970s survivors as they grow older.

Blackstone (1980) reported on the language status of three groups of at-risk children studied at 24 months of age. These groups consisted of low-birth-weight infants, full-term infants who manifested seizure disorders, and children of low birth weight who manifested seizure disorders. Children were evaluated using the *Denver Developmental Screening Test* (DDST) and a protocol to assess communication development. The results indicated a higher incidence of problems in the risk groups, when their performances were compared to available norm-referenced data. Nearly one-half of the infants with seizure disorders were severely handicapped. Most of the low-birth-weight children had normal DDST scores and normal neurological exams at 24 months, but their language status was judged by the speech-language clinician to be "questionable." The results from the group of children with low birth weights and seizures fell between the other two groups.

Blackstone argues that the questionable status of language abilities in these children, who otherwise have normal DDST exams, may reflect the kinds of language behaviors assessed at 2 years. The nature of the children's problems may be subtle. To assess children's language behavior, the *Sequenced Inventory of Communication Development* (SICD) and the *Receptive Expressive Emergent Language Scale* (REEL) were used. Correlation coefficients between a subject's performance at 2, 4, 6, 9, 12, and 18 months were compared to performance at 24 months. Neither the SICD nor the REEL test was useful in predicting performance in other than severely impaired children before 1 year of age; both tests were most predictive of 24-month scores at 18 months of age. Blackstone suggested a need to develop more sensitive developmental indices.

Hubatch, Johnson, Kistler, and Rutherford (1981) conducted a study of 10 low-birth-weight infants (780 to 1,730 grams) all of whom experienced respiratory-distress syndrome and required mechanical ventilation. These infants were compared to a group of 10 normal children matched for MLU. The premature children averaged 23 months of age and the normal children were 19 months old. All children were in the one-word stage. The premature children performed within normal limits on the Bayley Mental Development Index; the normal children did likewise on the DDST. Results indicated that the groups differed on measures of receptive and expressive language as well as in their developmental histories. The children with low birth weights and respiratory distress performed significantly more poorly in receptive vocabulary, and made fewer utterances. They also imitated less and said their first words later. Hubatch et al. state that the reason for differences was not known. They concluded that the group of children with low birth weight and respiratory-distress syndrome were "at-risk" for later communication disorders.

Findings of these studies of children born prematurely highlight some of the issues and limitations involved in attempting to predict language outcomes on the basis of antecedent conditions. Some of the issues are the following:

1. While advances in the medical care of children born prematurely have resulted in a reduction of catastrophic outcomes, there is variability in the developmental status of the children who survive. This makes it difficult to use the presence of an antecedent condition to identify children, since there exist problems of prediction secondary to the extended range of outcome possibilities.

2. Children born prematurely and who have had additional complications, such as asphyxia, respiratory-disease syndrome, or subependymal-intraventricular hemorrhage, may be at greater risk for language disorders. However, only longitudinal studies of the children and the individual varia-

tions in language acquisition and development will allow us to identify those genuinely at risk for later linguistic disorders.

3. Studies of children whose birth weights are less than 1,500 grams suggest that, for some, problems during the preschool years persist as disorders of reading and written language. However, the presence of later educational disorders in children with early language disorders is not restricted to children with low birth weight. The findings of later academic problems are similar to those reported on other groups of children, and these later studies have implicated early disruptions in speech and language development as precursors of later learning disabilities (Aram & Nation, 1980; Snyder, this volume; Strominger & Bashir, 1977).

4. The lack of appropriate measurements of early language behavior that can be useful as predictors of later language abilities makes the identification of children at risk for communication disorders difficult.

5. The historical presence of an antecedent condition alerts the clinician that the child may be at greater risk for later language disorder. However, because of variability in developmental outcomes, assessments of the child's cognitive and linguistic behavior is necessary to determine accurately the scope of the disabilities, and, therefore, the need for intervention. Miller (1982), in a consideration of etiology and language disorders, states that: "identifying the primary etiologic agent can predict an increased potential for language deficits, serving as an "at risk" register for language disorders [and as such can only] serve as a first level screen in early identification. . .(p. 64).

Review of these studies indicates the need for more precise information relating later speech and language outcomes to earlier perinatal and medical problems. Such documentation requires longitudinal studies ensuring an adequate understanding of neonatal complications and their impact on developmental language disorders. Further insights can be expected from the routine and periodic measures that would be taken of emerging speech and language during such longitudinal investigations. Additionally, comparable longitudinal data must be forthcoming on normal children developing language, so as to describe normal variability in the emergence of communication. We must move from a determination of at-risk-by-reference-to-antecedent conditions to a determination of at-risk-by-reference-to-indices-of-linguistic-and-communicative behaviors that have *predictive validity* for the later language status of the child.

Indices of Language Development: The Need

Clinicians' abilities to identify and to provide high quality service to children at risk are restricted by the lack of evaluation instruments that directly assess children's prelinguistic and early linguistic behaviors. We believe that the optimum way to develop indices for identification and assessment is through the study of the cognitive, affective, and linguistic status of the child, as well as the specific patterns of parent-child interaction that may affect the child's linguistic development.

Identification and assessment must incorporate a probabilistic perspective, since there presently are no clear clinical indices available that allow us to distinguish between children who demonstrate slow language development from those children who demonstrate "genuinely" altered language development. Leonard (1972) made the following comments concerning the probabilistic nature of early identification:

> The future linguistic behavior of children who use restricted utterances made up of early developing structures. . .proves difficult to predict. If such a child is three or older, it is not worth the risk of waiting to see whether his language develops further, for the social and educational developments in his near future will demand a more sophisticated linguistic system. And if the child is not yet three years of age? Many of us may not treat such a child because he may be a "late developer. " A few of us may recommend some sort of language intervention, but all of us are just guessing (p. 441).

The development of better assessment indices will increase the probability of identifying those children who are not at risk, those who are at risk for language disorder, and those who will require services. The need for what we call indices of language development results from seven considerations.

First, the measures designed for assessment of children whose language abilities are below the three-year level usually consist of a limited number of restricted tasks intended to do little more than assess major language milestones. For example, the *Receptive-Expressive Emergent Language Scale* (REEL) designed by Bzoch and League (1971) consists of a total of 66 items assessing receptive language and 66 items assessing expressive language. The test has three expressive items and three receptive items at each age interval, and extends across the range 3 months to 36 months. Age levels are divided into 2-; 3-; and 4-month intervals, so that six behaviors are assessed in each 3-month period. The *Preschool Language Scale* (revised form), another frequently used test, designed by Zimmerman, Steiner, and Evatt (1979), assesses children at 6-month intervals from 12 months to 7 years of age. This test contains only eight items at each age level, four measuring auditory comprehension and four measuring verbal abilities. The clinician has only eight different behaviors by which to reach a clinically competent decision, and to design a therapy plan. The *Reynell Developmental Language Scales* (Reynell, 1969) is probably one of the more sophisticated procedures and yet it too contains only a limited number of tasks for the assessment of any one stage of development. In addition, as Menyuk (1979) points out, many of the behaviors on standardized tests are difficult to quantify, e.g., how does one objectify "enjoys making sounds" or "combines sounds?" An analysis of the items of the *Denver Developmental Screening Test* allows the same conclusions (Miller, 1982).

Second, most assessment procedures are designed to obtain preliminary information about a child's language status; they cannot be used directly to prescribe the goals of intervention (Siegel, 1979). The clinician presently must rely on his or her own abilities to make a prescriptive determination. While clinicians engage in prescriptive determination, it is unclear that the results of their assessment allow them to direct intervention toward those aspects of language deficit that may best respond to environmental intervention (Menyuk & Wilbur, 1981). This is true because we are uncertain about which aspects of language behavior are influenced specifically by environmental factors. However, there are data that indicate a general compensatory or ameliorative influence of "good" home environments (see Siegel, 1982), and several studies that document the success of early intervention programs (Heber & Garber, 1975; Kysela, Hillyard, McDonald & Ahlsten-Taylor, 1981).

Third, the tasks included on currently available instruments assess discrete abilities not necessarily related to later linguistic accomplishments. Currently, we do not have the knowledge necessary to construct assessment instruments allowing for the specific assessments of earlier behaviors that serve as important precursors or predictors of the child's later linguistic development. For example, while we know that children produce increasingly diversified phonological units before the development of first words, we do not know how this phonological experimentation influences the emergence of first words or determines the course of later phonological development. Similarly, we do not know what earlier behaviors support the emergence of first words and what the influence of early acquisition of first words has on subsequent development of other linguistic and cognitive strategies.

Fourth, most assessment procedures do not measure language in terms of the interactive functions it serves for children and their communicative partners (McLean, 1979). Rees (1978) noted that current tests fail to explore the pragmatics of language. Moreover, such intervention efforts based on test results usually address only those abilities assessed, such as acquisition of vocabulary, development of syntax, and/or acquisition of speech sounds.

Fifth, since the currently available assessment instruments consist of a small number of items at each level, the clinician is limited in his or her ability to monitor effects of intervention. This issue can be addressed only by having an appraisal system that is sensitive to the changes occurring in the process of acquiring language. For example, the monitoring of the child's acquisition of a first lexicon should include some way of assessing both number and kind of words that the child knows as well as ways in which the child can use these words to communicate information, needs, and intent. Current assessment instruments do not provide this, since their principal goal is to determine if the child comprehends or produces a few commonly used object labels or actions.

Sixth, since a significant discrepancy from expectation must be present for the diagnosis of a language disorder to be made, intervention must wait until that significant difference has occurred. This is so because the determination of who is language impaired and who is not is based almost exclusively on the age at which the child accomplishes developmental milestones. Most often, clinicians use as a "rule of thumb" that the child must be a year behind in some or all aspects of language behavior. For a young child below the age of 3, this may mean that the child is not only a year behind before receiving assistance, but that the child has not mastered a significant proportion of language mastered by comparable peers. Therefore, a system of appraisal needs to be constructed examining component process as well as rate of emergence.

Seventh, while the role of the environment in the children's acquisition of language is receiving increasing attention in the literature on acquisition (Chapman, 1981; Furrow, Nelson, & Benedict, 1979; Snow & Ferguson, 1977), it is seldom considered in assessment. An exception to this can be seen in the work of those involved in the predictions of at-risk children. Sameroff and Chandler (1975) note that failures in the prediction of developmental disorders result from a lack of adequate knowledge regarding the complex and mutual influences between the child and the environment. These interactional influences serve to ameliorate or exacerbate the effects of earlier insults or trauma. Sameroff and Chandler conclude that developmental problems require developmental approaches for analysis. Cornell and Gottfried (1976) review some relevant studies of the ability of "stimulating" environments to compensate for developmental delay and for inadequate environments to increase delay.

Siegel (1982), in a recent study of 80 low-birth-weight children (birth weights less than 1,501 grams) and 68 full-term infants, attempted to increase the predictability of infant tests for assessing language and cognitive abilities using the Caldwell Inventory of Home Stimulation (HOME) (Elardo, Bradley, & Caldwell, 1975), along with the Uzgiris and Hunt Scale (1975) and the Bayley Infant Development Scales (1969). Children were assessed with the Bayley and Uzgiris-Hunt Scales at 4, 8, 12, and 18 months. The Caldwell Inventory was administered at 12 months of age. Outcome status was determined at two years of age by re-administering the Bayley Scales, the Hunt-Uzgiris Scales, and the Reynell Developmental Language Scales. Siegel found significant correlations between early measures and developmental outcomes particularly on certain subscales. She reported that children classified as being at risk in infancy, but who showed normal language and cognitive development at two years of age, came from families who scored higher on the HOME Scale. In contrast, children who were not classified as being at-risk in infancy, but who demonstrated later language or cognitive difficulty came from families who scored lower on the HOME Scale.

This type of data reinforces the need to include in assessment indices measures of the child's linguistic environment. Since at present we are unsure about the role of the environment in acquisition and its relation to developmental outcomes, here, too, we must be cautious. For example, Murphy (1982) studied phonetic development and mother responsiveness in a group of twelve children who differed in their rate of lexical acquisition. She found that the mothers' responsiveness to structured vocalizations (defined as vocalizations that contained at least one syllabic segment) did not influence strongly the rate of lexical acquisition. Mothers' responsiveness scores were higher for children whose lexical acquisition was more rapid than were mother's responsiveness scores for children whose lexicons developed more slowly. However, differences were minimized when the number of structured vocalizations were equated. Menyuk (1979), reviewing some of the results of mother-infant interaction studies, stated that perhaps only extreme variations in the amount and kind of speech provided by the caretaker will have an effect on the rate or quality of linguistic behaviors during the *early* years.

In reviewing studies of mothers' speech to children during the second year of life, Chapman (1981) suggested this stage as one in which the mother's verbal interaction with the child may play a differential role in development. She concluded that linguistically responsive—rather than linguistically stimulating—environments may accelerate acquisition. Longitudinal studies using appropriate assessment measures, and including outcome measures, should begin to yield *clinically* relevant answers to issues of environmental influence. We need to answer questions concerning matters like, "What is the mother responsive to?" and "What kinds of behavior in the child does her responsiveness affect?"—so that we may design more effective intervention programs.

What to Assess and How

This chapter began by describing an adult incantation for warding off white elephants. When we get down to the issue of what behaviors to assess and how, the white elephant problem becomes clearer. If the literature provided us with descriptions of linguistic differences between normally developing and impaired children, then the question of what, how, and when to measure would be simplified. This, however, is not the case. Johnston (1982) reviewed studies that attempted to find differences in syntax, grammatical morphology, relational semantics, lexical semantics, and pragmatics. She drew similar conclusions. Johnston stated that "research to date revealed virtually no consequence of learning language out of phase. Language disordered children may learn to speak slowly and late, but little else about their language has proved remarkable" (p. 789). The implication for assessment, and therefore prediction, appears to be that either we stop looking for differences or that we alter the way in which we attempt to isolate differences.

Johnston suggests that differences can be described perhaps by the simultaneous investigation of different aspects of linguistic behavior. As an example, she suggests that the appearance of inflectional morphemes such as progressive -*ing* and plural -*s* may accompany the production of complex rather than simple sentences in language-impaired children. It is interesting to note that as support for the above hypothesis, she cites four case studies which followed children longitudinally, rather than cross-sectional experimental investigations (Bax & Stevenson, 1977; Kerschensteiner & Huber, 1975; Trantham & Pederson, 1976; Weiner, 1974). Her own longitudinal work with Schery (Johnston & Schery, 1976) on the development of grammatical morphemes in language-impaired children, seems to support her hypothesis as well. She concluded that differences may appear once different aspects of the linguistic system are studied. To her suggestion, we would add that this research *should* be longitudinal, and that if prediction is a goal, follow-up analysis is necessary to determine the relations between earlier and later language behaviors.

The results of studying relations among different aspects of the grammar should advance our ability to define what constitutes a language disorder. Additionally, these studies should include the study of patterns of coherence and dissociation in linguistic, cognitive, and affective domains.

This approach may be critical for the objectification of the clinician's belief that many children who are language-impaired are different, not just delayed. The principal reason for this belief may derive from the fact that the clinician uses information from multiple domains. In general, during the course of assessment, clinicians focus simultaneously on the data from formal measurement of language abilities, on other data derived from their interactions with the child, and the family, historical information, and on data from other assessments. All of these sources allow the clinician to form hypotheses used directly in the diagnostic decision that a child is language-impaired. Indeed, the clinical diagnosis is based on information about the status of the child, and these data are derived by direct or observational information from at least three domains of behavior; for example, linguistic, cognitive, and affective.

Cross-domain research and studies of different aspects of the linguistic system appear to be a productive means for determining parameters of language impairment. We would like to offer an additional suggestion on how we might objectify clinical intuitions of difference. It would seem that time spent by a child within a stage must be included when matching children for linguistic development. Investigators (Leonard, 1979; Morehead & Ingram, 1973) have found that differences resulting from the analyses of children's production disappear when children are matched for MLU or Brown's stages of development, or both. Miller and Chapman (1981) investigated the relation between age and MLU in 123 normal-developing children between 17 and 59 months of age. Their children spent an average of 3.3 months in each of Brown's stages (ranges 3.1 to 3.9). We know it takes longer for language-impaired children to learn to speak, and that they may remain at a particular stage for a much longer time. It is possible, then, that when we match impaired children with children who move rapidly from stage to stage, we may be obscuring "time-in-stage differences" in results.

One potential design for investigating differences may be to match language impaired children with normal children when the language-impaired child has been in one of Brown's stages for a similar period of time. This means that both groups of children would need to be followed longitudinally until they have been in a stage for an equivalent amount of time. They would then be assessed at this point, (e.g., 2 months after their MLU had reached 2.0, but remained less than 2.5, if we use a change in MLU of 0.5 to indicate a change in stage). It would then be interesting to continue to follow these children using this same assessment procedure to describe the differences in the emerging patterns.

Another major issue facing those interested in assessment and prediction is the evaluation of age norms for the acquisition of certain language behaviors. Studies of different aspects of language acquisition show large variability, even among the normal population. Some examples may prove interesting. Menyuk (1978) describes the variability found in Brown's study of normally developing children (1973). Brown found that the age for achieving an MLS 2.5 was 25 to 30 months, for an MLU of 3.5 was 24 to 35 months, and for an MLU of 4.5 was 32 to 48 months. Menyuk found even wider discrepancies when she evaluated Morehead and Ingram's (1973) data on normal developing and developmentally dysphasic children. Whereas the normal children reached an MLU of 2-plus at 20 months of age, the dysphasic children did not reach this MLU until 60 months. This represents a difference of 40 months in age for attainment. The age discrepancy between the groups increased for attainment of an MLU of 5.5, the groups now differing by 71 months of age.

Nelson (1973) and Benedict (1979) report similar amounts of variability when studying normal children's acquisition of a first lexicon. For example, Nelson (1973) studied eighteen children and found that they reached a productive vocabulary of 50 words at an average age of 19.6 months, with a standard deviation of 2.89—but the range was 14 to 24 months. Benedict (1979) using a similar procedure with eight children, found a mean of 18.8 months and a range of 13 to 22 months. Reporting on the comprehension of 50 words, however, she found still smaller variability; that is, a mean age of 13.5 months, and a range of 10.2 to 16.5 months. If one were to presume that this small amount of data reflected the range seen in the normal population, one might conclude that it is reasonable to attempt to separate normal/at-risk children by acquisition rate. However, it would be necessary to determine the relation between lexical acquisition and other measures of language before one could determine accurately a ceiling score that could be used to determine the presence of a language disorder.

Hubbell (1981) expressed similar concern over age ranges provided by many standardized tests. He cited as one example the item in the *Denver Developmental Screening Test* that assesses comprehension of three prepositions. This item was passed by 25% of the children at 2.7 years, 50% at 3.1 years, 75% at 3.4 years, and 90% at 4.5 years. He concluded that these age ranges "encompass virtually half the children's total life span at the time the testing was done." The problem is to differentiate between children who are developing language normally, albeit at a slower rate, from those children who evidence altered acquisitional patterns that persist into the school years. It is likely that the relation between various aspects of language, or the *patterns* formed by different variables between groups at different developmental stages, may be more important than differences in rate.

A final issue that must be considered in the assessment and prediction of children with language impairments is how to evaluate the cognitive behaviors that have been identified as relating to language development (Bloom, 1970, 1973; Bowerman, 1974; Brown, 1973; Morehead & Ingram, 1973). Menyuk (1979) argued that some cognitive measures, for example, the *Bayley Scales of Infant Development,* are simply measuring limited aspects of linguistic development, rather than measuring cognitive development per se. Similarly, standardized performance tests that yield results showing language-impaired children operating within the "normal range" may not be measuring appropriate nonlinguistic behaviors. Many researchers have investigated cognitive functioning in language-impaired children and found that some of them appear to evidence nonlinguistic deficits (Brown, Redmond, Bass, Liebergott, & Swope, 1975; Folger & Leonard, 1978; Johnston & Ramstad, 1978; Lovell, Hoyle, & Siddall, 1968; Snyder, 1975). However, the developmental consequences of these nonlinguistic deficits remain speculative. Assessment and description of children's cognitive behavior may yield useful information for the content of therapy, but we have yet to determine the contribution made by nonlinguistic behavior to specific aspects of language acquisition.

There is a multitude of linguistic behaviors that can be used for constructing indices of language development (Miller, 1981; 1982). These behaviors have been discussed in the normal-language-acquisition literature, and a few have been investigated in children with language impairments. The usefulness of these measures (i.e., behaviors across linguistic domains) for predicting later language development cannot be discussed at this time because outcome studies have yet to be done.

In summary, to construct indices of language development for the identification and assessment of children at risk for language disorders, we will need to engage in:

1. Longitudinal study of larger groups of normal children, as well as subgroups of language-impaired children.

2. Measurement of children's linguistic behavior that allows for simultaneous investigation of different aspects of linguistic behavior.

3. Studies of patterns of coherence and dissociation in linguistic, cognitive, and affective domains.

4. Studies of the relation between earlier and later language ability as they relate to linguistic and school outcomes.

Those interested in pursuing the construction of clinically useful assessment procedures must be prepared for the constraints of such research. They will need to face the reliability and validity issues described above.

They will need to find methods for dealing with the variability in language acquisition they will inevitably find. While group trends may be a sufficient first approximation, the final question relates to the single child and the determination of his or her needs. The issues are important.

Acknowledgements

This work was supported in part by grant number G008006727 from the Office of Special Education and Rehabilitative Services, U.S. Department of Education, to M.C. Schultz. The authors gratefully acknowledge the additional support of the Esther S. and Joseph M. Shapiro Center for Research in Communicative Disorders and the Hazel Moore Graves Memorial Fund.

References

Aram, D.M., & Nation, J.E. Preschool language disorders and subsequent language and academic difficulties. *Journal of Communication Disorders,* 1980, *13,* 159-170.

Bax, M., & Stevenson, P. Analysis of a developmental language delay. *Proceedings of the Royal Society of Medicine,* 1977, *70,* 727-728.

Bayley, N. *Bayley Scales of Infant Development.* New York: Psychological Corporation, 1969.

Benedict, H. Early lexical development: Comprehension and production. *Journal of Child Language,* 1979, *6,* 183-200.

Blackstone, S.W. *Communication assessment of high risk infants.* Unpublished doctoral dissertation, University of Pittsburgh, 1980.

Bloom, L. *Language development: Form and function in emerging grammars.* Cambridge, MA: MIT Press, 1970.

Bloom, L. *One word at a time.* The Hague: Mouton, 1973.

Bowerman, M. Discussion summary—development of concepts underlying language. In R.L. Schiefelbusch & L.L. Lloyd (Eds.), *Language perspectives—Acquisition, retardation, and intervention.* Baltimore: University Park Press, 1974.

Brown, J., Redmond, A., Bass, K., Liebergott, J.W., & Swope, S., *Symbolic play in normal and language-impaired children.* Paper presented at the Annual Convention of the American Speech and Hearing Association, Washington, D.C., November, 1975.

Brown, R. *A first language: The early stages.* Cambridge, MA: Harvard University Press, 1973.

Bzoch, R., & League, R. *Assessing language skills in infancy.* Gainsville, FL: Tree of Life Press, 1971.

Cairns, G.F., & Butterfield, E.C. Assessing language-related skills of prelinguistic children. *Allied Health and Behavioral Sciences,* 1981, *1,* 81-130.

Chapman, R.S. Mother-child interaction in the second year of life. In R. Schiefelbusch & D.D. Bricker (Eds.), *Early language: Acquisition and intervention.* Baltimore: University Park Press, 1982.

Cornell, E.H., & Gottfried, A.W. Intervention with premature infants. *Child Development,* 1976, *47,* 32-39.

DeHirsch, K., Jansky, J., & Langford, W.S. The oral language performance of premature children and controls. *Journal of Speech and Hearing Disorders,* 1964, *29,* 60-69.

Ehrlich, C.H., Shapiro, E., Kimball, B., & Huttner, M. Communication skills in five-year-old children with high risk neonatal histories. *Journal of Speech and Hearing Research,* 1973, *16,* 522-529.

Elardo, R., Bradley, R.H., & Caldwell, B.M. The relation of infants' home environments to mental tests performance from six to thirty-six months: A longitudinal analysis. *Child Development,* 1975, *46,* 71-76.

Field, T. Interaction patterns of preterm and term infants. In T. Field, A.M. Sostek, S. Goldberg, & H. Shuman (Eds.), *Infants born at risk: Behavior and development.* New York: Spectrum Publications, 1979.

Fitzhardinge, P. Current outcome: ICU populations. In A.W. Brann & J.J. Volpe (Eds.), *Neonatal neurological assessment and outcome.* Columbus, OH: Ross Laboratories, 1980.

Fitzhardinge, P.M. & Ramsay, M. The improving outlook for the small prematurely born infant. *Developmental Medicine and Child Neurology,* 1973, *15,* 447-459.

Folger, M., & Leonard, L.B. Language and sensorimotor development during the early period of referential speech. *Journal of Speech and Hearing Research,* 1978, *21,* 519-527.

Furrow, D., Nelson, K., & Benedict, H. Mothers' speech to children and synthetic development: Some simple relationships. *Journal of Child Language,* 1979, *6,* 423-442.

Heber, R., & Garber, H. The Milwaukee project: A study of the use of family intervention to prevent cultural-familial retardation. In B. Friedlander, G. Steritt, & S. Kirk (Eds.) *Exceptional infant,* (Vol. 1). New York: Brunner/Mazel, 1975.

Hubatch, L.M., Johnson, C.J., Kistler, D.J., & Rutherford, D.R. *Language development of high risk infants.* Paper presented at the Annual Convention of the American Speech-Language-Hearing Association, Los Angeles, November, 1981.

Hubbel, R. *Children's language disorders: An integrated approach.* Englewood Cliffs, NJ: Prentice-Hall, 1981.

Johnston, J. The language disordered child. In N.A. Lass, L.V. McReynolds, J.L. Northern, & D.E. Yoder (Eds.), *Speech, language and hearing, Vol. II. Pathologies of Speech and Language.* Philadelphia: W.B. Saunders, 1982.

Johnston, J., & Ramstad, V. Cognitive development in preadolescent language-impaired children. In M. Burns & J. Andrews (Eds.), *Selected papers in language and phonology.* Evanston, IL: Institute for continuing Professional Education, 1978.

Johnston, J., & Schery, T. The use of grammatical morphemes by children with communication disorders. In D. Morehead & A. Morehead (Eds.), *Normal and deficient child language.* Baltimore: University Park Press, 1976.

Kastein, S., & Fowler, E.P. Language development among survivors of premature birth. *Archives of Otolaryngology,* 1959, *69,* 131-135.

Kerschensteiner, M., & Huber, W. Grammatical impairment in developmental aphasia. *Cortex,* 1975, *11,* 264-282.

Kitchen, W.H., Ryan, M.M., Rickards, A., McDougall, A.B., Billson, F.A., Keir, E.H., & Naylor, F.D. A longitudinal study of very low birthweight infants. IV: An overview of performance at eight years of age. *Developmental Medicine and Child Neurology,* 1980, *22,* 172-188.

Koops, B.L. & Harmon, R.J. Studies on long-term outcome in newborns with birthweights under 1,500 grams. *Advances in behavioral pediatrics* (Vol. 1). New York: JAI press, 1980.

Kysela, G., Hillyard, A., McDonald, L., & Ahlsten-Taylor, J. Early intervention: Design and evaluation. In R. Schiefelbusch & D. Bricker (Eds.), *Early language intervention.* Baltimore: University Park Press, 1981.

Lassman, F.M., Fisch, R.O., Vetter, D.K., & LaBenz, E.S. *Early correlates of speech, language and hearing: The collaborative perinatal project of the national institute of neurological and communicative disorders and stroke.* Littleton, MA: PSG Publishing, 1980.

Leonard, L.B. What is language deviant? *Journal of Speech and Hearing Disorders,* 1972, *37,* 427-446.

Leonard, L.B. Language impairment in children. *Merrill-Palmer Quarterly,* 1979, *25,* 205-232.

Lovell, K., Hoyle, H., & Siddall, M. A study of some aspects of the play and language of young children with delayed speech. *Journal of Child Psychology and Psychiatry,* 1968, *9,* 41-50.

Lubchenco, L.O. *The high risk infant.* Philadelphia: W.B. Saunders, 1976.

McLean, J.E. Sequenced inventory of communication development. In F.L. Darley (Ed.), *Evaluation of appraisal techniques in speech and language pathology.* Reading, MA: Addison-Wesley Publishing, 1979.

Menyuk, P. Linguistic problems in children with developmental dysphasia. In M. Wyke (Ed.), *Developmental dysphasia.* London: Academic Press, 1978.

Menyuk, P. Methods used to measure linguistic competence during the first five years of life. In R.B. Kearsley & I.E. Sigel (Eds.), *Infants at risk: Assessment of cognitive functioning.* Hillsdale, NJ: Lawrence Erlbaum Associates, 1979.

Menyuk, P., & Wilbur, R. Preface to special issue on language disorders. *Journal of Autism and Developmental Disorders,* 1981, 11.

Miller, J. *Assessing language production in children.* Baltimore: University Park Press, 1981.

Miller, J.F. Identifying children with language disorders and describing their language performance. In J. Miller, D.E. Yoder, & R. Schiefelbusch (Eds.), *Contemporary issues in language intervention.* Rockville, MD: The American Speech-Language-Hearing Association, 1982.

Miller, J.F., & Chapman, R.S. The relation between age and mean length of utterance in morphemes. *Journal of Speech and Hearing Research,* 1981, *24,* 154-161.

Morehead, D.M., & Ingram, D. The development of base syntax in normal and linguistically deviant children. *Journal of Speech and Hearing Research,* 1973, *16,* 330-352.

Murphy, R.L. *Predicting lexical acquisition.* Unpublished master's thesis, Emerson College, 1982.

Nelson, K. Structure and strategy in learning to talk. *Monographs of the society for research in child development,* No. 149, 1973.

Pillitteri, A. *Maternal-newborn nursing.* Boston: Little, Brown & Co., 1981.

Ramey, C.T., Trohanis, P.L., & Hostler, S.L. An introduction. In C.T. Ramey & P.L. Trohanis (Eds.), *Finding and educating high-risk and handicapped infants.* Baltimore: University Park Press, 1982.

Rees, N.S. Pragmatics of language: Applications to normal and disordered language development. In R. Schiefelbusch (Ed.), *Bases of language intervention.* Baltimore: University Park Press, 1978.

Reynell, J. *Reynell Developmental Language Scales.* Windsor, Eng.: NFER Publishing, 1969.

Sameroff, A.J., & Chandler, M.J. Reproductive risk and the continuum of caretaking causality. In J. D. Horowitz (Ed.), *Review of child development research* (Vol. 4). Chicago: University of Chicago Press, 1975.

Siegel, G.M. Appraisal of language development. In F.L. Darley (Ed.), *Evaluation of appraisal techniques in speech and language pathology.* Reading, MA.: Addison-Wesley Publishing, 1979.

Siegel, L.S. Reproductive, perinatal and environmental factors as predictors of the cognitive and language development of preterm and full-term infants. *Child Development,* 1982, *53,* 963-973.

Snow, C.E., & Ferguson, C.A. *Talking to children: Language input and acquisition.* Cambridge, Eng.: Cambridge University Press, 1977.

Snyder, L. *Pragmatics in language disabled children: Their prelinguistic and early verbal performances and presuppositions.* Unpublished doctoral dissertation, University of Colorado, 1975.

Stewart, A.L., & Reynolds, E.O. Improved prognosis for infants of very low birth weight. *Pediatrics,* 1974, *34,* 724-735.

Strominger, A., & Bashir, A. *A nine-year follow-up of language disordered children.* Paper presented at the Annual Convention of the American Speech-Language-Hearing Association, Chicago, November, 1977.

Thompson, T., & Reynolds, J. Neonatal intensive care. *Journal of Perinatal Medicine,* 1977, *5,* 59-75.

Tjossem, T.D. Early intervention: Issues and approaches. In T.D. Tjossem (Ed.), *Intervention strategies for high risk infants and young children.* Baltimore: University Park Press, 1976.

Trantham, C.R., & Pederson, J. *Normal language development.* Baltimore: Williams & Wilkins, 1976.

Uzgiris, I.C., & Hunt, J.M. *Assessment in infancy: Ordinal scales of psychological development.* Urbana, IL: University of Illinois Press, 1975.

Weiner, P. A language delayed child at adolescence. *Journal of Speech and Hearing Disorders,* 1974, *34,* 302-312.

Zimmerman, I., Steiner, V., & Evatt, R. *Preschool language scale.* Columbus, OH: Charles E. Merrill, 1979.

Jon F. Miller
Thomas F. Campbell
Robin S. Chapman
Susan E. Weismer

Language Behavior in Acquired Childhood Aphasia

Most children learn to talk easily and rapidly despite variation in environment and endowment. Among the exceptions are children with mental deficiency, hearing impairment, central-nervous-system impairment affecting the speech production mechanism, emotional disturbance, or extreme environmental deprivation. For these children, the cause of the language deficit is evident. Another group of children, for no identified reason, begins the language-acquisition process late and progresses more slowly and with more difficulty than their peers. These children have been variously labeled developmentally aphasic, dysphasic, language-impaired, language-disabled, and language-disordered (Johnston, 1982; Leonard, 1979). The children in this latter group are considered to have developmental disorders specific to language learning that result in significant rate differences for at least some aspects of the language system.

Acquired Childhood Aphasia

This chapter is about yet another group of children, who differ from all the preceding groups in that they start out learning language normally, achieving developmental milestones at the appropriate rate. Their progress is disturbed as a direct result of neurological impairment. A variety of etiologies are associated with this group, including cerebral trauma, head tumors, cerebrovascular abnormalities, and seizure disorders. These children have acquired language disorders and are generally refered to as *acquired aphasics*.

© College-Hill Press, Inc. All rights, including that of translation, reserved. No part of this publication may be reproduced without the written permission of the publisher.

Within this group of acquired childhood aphasics is a group whose language disturbance is accompanied by a seizure disorder and/or abnormal electroencephalographic (EEG) findings (Landau & Kleffner, 1957). These children have increasingly been the subject of investigation, particularly case reports (e.g., Campbell, 1982; Cromer, 1981; Deonna, Fletcher, & Voumard, in press). The cases available in the literature are quite diverse in presenting symptoms, degree of pathology, course, resolution, and outcome of the neurological and language deficit. The onset of the disorder may be gradual or acute, with deficits lasting from a few days to years. Some children have been reported to recover completely, some remain the same, and others display progressive disorders (Mantovani & Landau, 1980).

These cases provide a unique opportunity for studies that improve our understanding of deficits associated with a particular diagnosed neurological impairment in the developmental period. A detailed review of this literature will provide insight into the complexity of this disorder, and the theoretical and clinical issues raised in determining prognosis and constructing behavioral and medical intervention programs. Of special interest in this chapter will be the linguistic outcomes of the various onset, severity, and descriptive characteristics associated with acquired aphasia accompanied by seizure disorders.

Acquired Childhood Aphasia
Secondary to a Convulsive Disorder

Landau and Kleffner (1957) originally reported examples of acquired aphasia associated with a convulsive disorder and paroxysmal EEG abnormalities. They described five children, ages five to nine years, who displayed both receptive and expressive language deficits following a normal period of speech and language development. The regression in these children's language abilities was either accompanied, preceded, or followed by seizures and other neurological manifestations. In some, the onset of the syndrome was noted to be gradual, while in others it was sudden. Improvement of speech and language skills in one child occurred with no intervention whatsoever; however, in four cases, improvement was aided by medication for seizures and language intervention. Their case reports included little information regarding specific speech and language behaviors displayed before, during, or following the disorder.

In the twenty-five years since Landau and Kleffner's first report, case studies have followed that have added fragmentary information to this puzzling clinical disorder. Twenty-six published articles describing the disorder have verified many of Landau and Kleffner's original observations. Still, virtually no data have been presented in recent years to provide new insight into the mechanisms underlying the neurological and language dysfunctions. Description of this population of children as reported in the literature follows.

Sex

Tables 3-1 through 3-3 present a review of the 94 cases of this syndrome reported in the literature. Examination of Table 3-1 reveals that in the 75 cases which present gender data, males were affected 65% of the time. The overall ratio of approximately two males to every female has also been reported in an earlier review by Cooper and Ferry (1978).

Time and Rate of Onset

Time of onset ranges from 1-1/2 to 13 years. Deonna, Beaumanoir, Gaillard, and Assal (1977) note that most of these children experience initial language loss between the ages of 3 and 7 years. In 25% of the cases reviewed (Table 3-1), the onset of the language regression was gradual, occurring over a period of longer than six months. In the remainder, language loss was more abrupt. In some cases, it occurred within a matter of hours or days. Language use during the early phases of this disorder has frequently been characterized as fluctuating, with performance varying widely across days or within a day.

Neurological Characteristics

Aside from the seizure (EEG abnormalities were the basis for case selection), the clinical neurological examination for these children was essentially normal. One case of flattening of the lower face, facial apraxia, and incoordination and clumsiness was reported (Gascon, Victor, Lombroso, & Goodglass, 1973; Landau & Kleffner, 1957). As indicated in Table 3-2, all cases that reported EEG results (84) revealed abnormal electrical discharges from one or both temporal lobes.

Of the 68 children who displayed some type of seizure (general, psychomotor, myoclonic, minor motor, petit mal, or complex partial), 43% experienced seizures before the dysphasia, 16% displayed co-occurrence of seizures and language regression, and 41% reported the language disorder to have occurred before onset of the seizures. Language regression in this final group of children has been noted to have occurred from six months (Shoumaker, Bennett, Bray, & Curless, 1974) to two years (Gascon et al., 1973) before onset of seizures.

Table 3-1
Sex, time, and rate of onset characteristics reported in 26 studies of acquired childhood aphasia secondary to a convulsive disorder. (NR = no report)

Author	N	Sex		Time of Onset			
		Male	Female	Age, yrs.	6 mos.	6 mos.	6 mos.
Landau & Kleffner (1957)	5	2	3	3.5-9		2	3
Barlow (1968)	1	1	0	8.5		NR	NR
Stein & Curry (1968)	1	0	1	2.6		0	1
Worster-Drought (1971)	14	5	9	3-7		0	14
Gascon, Victor, Lombroso, & Goodglass (1973)	3	3	0	3.5-6		2	1
Harel, Walsh, & Menkes (1973)	1	1	0	3		NR	NR
Deuel & Lenn (1974)	3	NR	NR	NR		NR	NR
Huskisson (1974)	1	1	1	4.10		0	1
McKinney & McGreal (1974)	9	6	3	3-13		NR	NR
Shoumaker, Bennett, Bray, & Curless (1974)	3	3	0	5-6		1	2
Lou, Brandt, & Bruhn (1977)	4	2	2	3.4		3	1
Deonna, Beaumanoir, Gaillard, & Assal (1977)	6	5	1	3.5-9		1	5

Study						
Deuel & Lenn (1977)	1	0	1	4	1	0
Rapin, Mattis, Rowan, & Golden (1977)	3	3	0	1.5-3	0	3
Campbell & Heaton (1978)	1	1	0	5	1	0
Cooper & Ferry (1978)	3	3	0	2.5-10	0	3
Koepp & Lagenstein (1978)	1	1	0	4.5	0	1
Kracke (1978)	7	NR	NR	3-5	NR	NR
van Harskamp, van Dongen, & Loonen (1978)	1	0	1	4	0	1
Jordan (1980)	1	1	0	5	NR	NR
Mantovani & Landau (1980)	3	1	2	3-6	2	1
de Negri (1980)	8	NR	NR	3-6	NR	NR
Deonna, Fletcher, & Voumard (in press)	1	1	0	2.5	0	1
Waisman Study (1981)	6	5	1	2.5-7	4	2
Holmes & McKeever (1981)	2	NR	NR	NR	NR	NR
Campbell (1982)	5	4	1	2.5-8	0	5
Totals	**94**	**49**	**26**	**1.5-13**	**17**	**45**

Table 3-2
Seizure status in 26 studies of acquired childhood aphasia secondary to a conculsive disorder.
(NR = no report)

Author	Abnormal			Seizures Precede Aphasia	Co-occur	Aphasia Precedes Seizures
	N	EEG	Seizures			
Landau & Kleffner (1957)	5	5	5	4	0	1
Barlow (1968)	1	1	1	1	0	0
Stein & Curry (1968)	1	1	1	NR	NR	NR
Worster-Drought (1971)	14	14	14	NR	NR	NR
Gascon et al. (1973)	3	3	3	1	1	1
Harel et al. (1973)	1	1	1	0	0	1
Deuel & Lenn (1974)	3	NR	NR	NR	NR	NR
Huskisson (1974)	1	1	NR	NR	NR	NR
McKinney & McGreal (1974)	9	9	7	4	0	3
Shoumaker et al. (1974)	3	3	2	0	0	2
Lou et al. (1977)	4	4	3	2	1	0
Deonna et al. (1974)	6	6	5	2	1	2
Deuel & Lenn (1977)	1	1	1	1	0	0
Rapin et al. (1977)	3	3	2	0	0	2

Campbell & Heaton (1978)	3	1	1	0	0	1
Cooper & Ferry (1978)	3	3	3	0	2	1
van Harskamp et al. (1978)	1	1	1	0	0	1
Jordan (1980)	1	1	1	NR	NR	NR
Kracke (1978)	7	NR	NR	NR	NR	NR
Koepp & Lagenstein (1978)	1	1	0	0	0	0
Mantovani & Landau (1980)	3	3	0	0	0	0
de Negri (1980)	8	8	6	NR	NR	NR
Deonna, et al. (in press)	1	1	NR	NR	NR	NR
Waisman Study (1981)	6	6	6	3	1	2
Holmes & McKeever (1981)	2	2	2	NR	NR	NR
Campbell (1982)	5	5	3	1	1	1
Totals	**94**	**84**	**68**	**19**	**7**	**18**

Audiological Characteristics

Because the language disorder typically includes disturbance of comprehension as well as production skills, the children often give the impression of having become deaf. Those studies that do include audiological information, however, typically indicate normal hearing sensitivity for pure tones throughout the entire frequency range. Normal early components of auditory-evoked potentials have also revealed normal hearing sensitivity in several cases (Gascon et al., 1973). Speech audiometric tests are often not attempted in light of the severe receptive and expressive language deficit. Waters (1974) cautions that interpretation of any behavioral audiological test may present problems.

Behavioral Characteristics

Behavioral abnormalities have been frequently noted in this population of children (Campbell & Heaton, 1978; Deonna et al., 1977; Deuel & Lenn, 1977; Gascon et al., 1973; Shoumaker et al., 1974; Stein & Curry, 1968). Behaviors such as inattention, withdrawal, aggressiveness, temper outbursts, refusing to respond, and, in some cases, hyperactivity, have been observed. Mantovani and Landau (1980) speculated that behavioral problems in this group of children "may reflect a primary disinhibition at limbic or diencephalic levels" (p. 528). It is equally likely, however, that such behaviors may be secondary reactions to the sudden loss in communication abilities. This interpretation is supported by the fact that many of these behaviors disappear once the child is provided with an alternative communication system (Campbell & Heaton, 1979). Deonna et al. (1977) note that "a bizarre, sudden, or insidious onset or language regression in a previously normal child, with no other evidence of organic illness, can easily be mistaken for a psychiatric reaction" (p. 272).

Cognitive Characteristics

Of the 72 cases that provide results of cognitive testing, over 85% show normal intellectual functioning, as indicated by a nonverbal performance IQ score of 90 or above, assessed with a variety of nonverbal measures. Comparable measures prior to seizures or language loss, however, have not been available. The difference between verbal and nonverbal cognitive abilities can vary considerably. In their discussion of nine adult cases who were followed up 10 or more years after onset of the disorder, Mantovani and Landau (1980) found a discrepancy of 12 to 15 points between verbal and performance scores on the Wechsler Adult Intelligence Scale (WAIS).

Language Characteristics

All 94 review cases displayed both receptive and expressive language deficits. Waters (1974), Campbell and Heaton (1978) and Jordan (1980), among others, report that difficulties in auditory comprehension appear first, followed by expressive speech and language difficulties. Communication problems recur or persist beyond six months in 94% of the cases (see Table 3-3). Reports from parents reveal that these children do not carry out verbal commands which they could perform previously, and, in certain respects, give the appearance of being deaf. For one 9-year-old male reported by Campbell and Heaton (1978), spoken commands were responded to by puzzled expressions and a shoulder shrug, or the commands were ignored completely. Worster-Drought (1971), in a review of 14 children, found that some were capable of understanding simple commands, while others appeared to be almost oblivious to verbal stimuli. The child reported by Stein and Curry (1968) comprehended better when visual cues were used to enhance spoken language; however, even when lip-reading cues were made available, comprehension remained poor. Campbell and Heaton (1979) reported that reading comprehension abilities displayed by their children were often far in advance of their ability to comprehend speech. Spontaneous speech, in particular, poses major comprehension problems for many of these individuals. For example, a 15-year-old boy, whose speech and language eventually returned to normal, stated that connected speech sounded like "blah, blah, blah" to him (Landau & Kleffner, 1957).

In addition to deficits in comprehension of speech, auditory receptive problems have also been observed in discriminating and recognizing nonspeech sounds (Stein & Curry, 1968; Campbell & Heaton, 1978).

Expressively, some children became totally mute. Some use jargon-like speech characterized by isolated production of consonants or vowels. And, in many cases, they resort to gestures and grunts. Others display a variety of misarticulations, inappropriate substitutions of words, and word-retrieval problems. One child, who subsequently improved, said that he understood what was said to him, but could not recall the words he wanted to say (Landau & Kleffnner, 1957).

Voice quality is affected in some children. Worster-Drought (1971) and Cooper and Ferry (1978) report that some children retain normal quality and suprasegmental characteristics, while others shift to a high fundamental frequency lacking normal inflection. Their speech is similar to that of deaf children. Results of instrumental assessments of voice quality and suprasegmental characteristics have not been reported. Nor does the literature contain precise descriptions of these children's articulatory, phonological, syntactic, or semantic systems.

Table 3-3
Duration of language disorder reported in 26 studies of acquired
aphasia secondary to a convulsive disorder.

		Duration of Language Deficit		
	N	*<6 mo.*	*>6 mo.*	*Recur*
Landau & Kleffner (1957)	5	0	3	2
Barlow (1968)	1	0	1	0
Stein & Curry (1968)	1	0	1	0
Worster-Drought (1971)	14	0	14	0
Gascon et al. (1973)	3	0	2	1
Harel et al. (1973)	1	0	1	0
Deuel & Lenn (1974)	3	0	3	0
Huskisson (1974)	1	0	1	0
McKinney & McGreal (1974)	9	3	6	0
Shoumaker et al. (1974)	3	0	2	1
Lou et. al. (1977)	4	1	3	0
Deonna et al. (1977)	6	0	5	1
Deuel & Lenn (1977)	1	0	0	1
Rapin et al. (1977)	3	0	3	0
Campbell & Heaton (1978)	1	0	0	1
Cooper & Ferry (1978)	3	0	3	0
Kracke (1978)	7	0	7	0
Koepp & Lagenstein (1978)	1	0	1	0
van Harskamp et al. (1978)	1	0	1	0
Jordan (1980)	1	0	0	1
Mantovani & Landau (1980)	3	0	3	0
de Negri (1980)	8	NR	NR	NR
Deonna et al. (1981)	1	1	0	0
Waisman Study (1981)	6	0	6	0
Holmes & McKeever (1981)	2	0	2	0
Campbell (1982)	5	0	3	2
Totals	**94**	**5**	**71**	**10**

(NR = no report)

Relationship Among EEG, Seizures, and Language Deficit

The relationships among the EEG disturbance, seizures, and the language disorder have not been clearly demonstrated. However, Mantovani and Landau (1980) stated that

> our data do not indicate that the absence of seizures is a decisive factor for therapeutic response or ultimate outcome. Until more is known about pathogenesis, we prefer to continue the original designation, because we believe that paroxysmal EEG is the pathophysiologic definition of convulsive disorder (p. 528).

Landau and Kleffner (1957) originally adopted a similar point of view when they stated: "The seizure manifestations have been readily controlled medically and are not closely correlated with the aphasic symtoms. In all cases a severe paroxysmal electroencephalographic abnormality, usually diffuse, is observed" (p. 530).

The nature of the relationship of the EEG disturbance to the language disorder, however, remains ambiguous. Landau and Kleffner (1957) noted that "electroencephalographic improvement tended to parallel improvement in speech re-education" (p. 530). Shoumaker et al., (1974) also reported that improvement in speech correlated with a decrease in the abnormalities on the EEG. In all three of the patients observed by Shoumaker and colleagues, the greatest spike-wave discharges were noted when the language disorder was at its peak; and language improvement was not observed until the abnormal electrical activity had disappeared. They further stated that improvement in speech/language functioning was not sudden once the discharges decreased, and, in one case, it lagged for 2 to 3 months. Rose (1969), in fact, noted that recovery of speech/language skills (not further specified) may lag behind EEG improvement up to 6 months.

Conversely, Worster-Drought (1971) and Rapin, Mattis, Rowan, and Golden, (1977) have reported persistent speech and language problems despite subsequent normal EEGs. In addition, Campbell and Heaton (1978) describe a boy who suddenly acquired a severe speech and language deficit after 5 years of normal language development. Medical reports revealed that the child presented normal EEG tracings 2 months after the onset of the disorder, but language skills never returned to normal. As can be surmised from these few studies, the relationship between the EEG disturbance and the language disorder remains unclear, and is likely to remain so until more is known about the cause of the disorder.

Pathogenesis

Deonna, Beaumanoir, Gaillard, and Assal (1977) suggest that the variability in these children's recovery of speech and language abilities may relate to differing pathogeneses. Although data to support such a notion are not available, several hypotheses have been proposed. Landau and Kleffner (1957) discuss the possibility that regression in speech and language skills may result from the functional ablation of the primary cortical language areas by persistent electrical discharges in these regions. This hypothesis is supported by Sato and Dreifuss (1972), who posit that the language regression in one child was due to continuous bilateral synchronous temporal spike activity, which caused a dysfunction of both hemispheres.

Gascon et al. (1973, p. 162) state that "EEG discharges are a cortical manifestation of a lower level subcortical de-afferenting process." This hypothesis implies that the electrical discharges displayed by these children are a secondary factor, and are not directly responsible for the aphasia. These authors suggest that there is some subcortical involvement of the auditory pathways. However, case reports reveal normal hearing- and auditory-evoked response profiles in some of these children (Campbell, 1982; Waisman Study, 1981), indicating integrity of the auditory pathways. Such cases argue against the hypothesis.

Gascon et al. (1973) further speculate that the cause of the disorder might be some pathogenetic mechanism that is related in an unknown way to the convulsive disorder. Deonna et al. (1977) suggest that these children may have an "unusual genetic or acquired pattern of cerebral organization which renders them particularly sensitive to brain damage or seizure activity as far as language is concerned" (p. 271).

Pathoanatomical studies to support these hypotheses are limited. McKinney and McGreal (1974) examined brain tissue taken from one child. No abnormalities were noted. However, they believe that the fluctuating course in many of these patients indicates an inflammatory mechanism. This follows Worster-Drought's (1971) hyphothesis that there is an active low-grade selective encephalitis which affects the temporal lobes. Results from a cortical biopsy reported by Lou, Brandt, and Bruhn (1977) clearly showed inflammation of the meninges with leukocyte infiltration and thickening. The results also revealed gliosis and loss of neurons, suggesting a meningoencephalities of the "slow virus" type. Rasmussen and McCann (1968) report similar findings in adults with prolonged temporal lobe seizures.

If an inflammatory process were localized in the region of the temporal lobe, it certainly could result in both language dysfunction and seizures. However, additional pathoanatomical investigations suggest other possible causes. Rapin et al. (1977) found a small vascular anomaly in the left angular gyrus of one of these children. In a second child, they found diminished vascularization in the area of the left middle cerebral artery.

Interpretation of these findings is limited because there have been no occasions for pathoanatomic studies close in time to symptom onset. Until noninvasive means of assessing cortical structure and function are better developed, the true cause and nature of the syndrome will remain a matter of speculation.

Prognosis

The long-term course of the disorder remains unclear. Several researchers (most notably Gascon et al., 1973; Landau & Kleffner, 1957; Mantovani & Landau, 1980; Rapin et al., 1977; Worster-Drought, 1971) have reported a number of children who regained normal receptive and expressive language skills following their sudden loss. A review of the reported cases, however, indicates that more than 80% of the children display both receptive and expressive language deficits that persist longer than 6 months. According to Gascon et al. (1973), the degree of residual language loss ranges from verbal-auditory agnosia with no verbal communication, to mild deficits in academic areas such as spelling and reading. In a survey of 45 case studies, Cooper and Ferry (1978) reported that 42% of the children were left with a severe auditory-comprehension deficit, 24% had moderate-to-mild deficits, and 33% made a complete recovery. The explanation for this variability in recovery remains one of the most puzzling features of the disorder.

Grouping according to the limited descriptive data available does not appear to simplify prognosis. Based on general clinical features (onset characteristics, number of seizures, and the course of the language disorder), Deonna et al. (1977) propose three different clinical varieties of the syndrome.

One group consists of those children in whom language development is abruptly interrupted in association with seizures. The language deficit persists for variable amounts of time (anywhere from a few days to several years) and Deonna et al. (1977) suggest that the recovery is "too rapid to be explained by a shift in speech dominance" (p. 270). They further suggest that the language disorder may represent "a functional disconnection of language mechanisms without any newly acquired lesion" (p. 270).

The second group includes children who show little or no improvement in verbal communication skills after a major seizure, or following repeated episodes of language fluctuation. Recovery for these children, when it occurs, has been reported to take place in the course of months or years. Deonna et al. speculate that if recovery does take place, one might assume that the other hemisphere has "taken over speech." Limited empirical data are available to support this speculation.

The third group concerns those children who gradually develop a moderate-to-severe deficit in auditory comprehension. Children in this group may experience few or no seizures, and, often, appear to be deaf. Variable degrees of recovery have been reported in this group of children. In many cases, little improvement has been reported after several years.

These three groups, constructed on the basis of differing types of onset (sudden, fluctuating, or gradual) and presence or absence of seizures, each display varying rates and degrees of recovery. It remains unclear whether the language abilities of the children within each group were homogeneous in nature. Thus, grouping by onset characteristics does not appear to create groups more homogeneous in prognosis.

Illustrations of New Directions for Research

As the preceding summary makes clear, children with acquired aphasia associated with convulsive disorders show a variety of patterns of onset and recovery. The language disorder may itself be the earliest symptom of central-nervous-system disease, and the last to recover, if recovery takes place at all. How is the clinician to predict the course of recovery and make recommendations for treatment in the face of this variability in patterns of onset and recovery? One promising direction for new research, we believe, comes from a far more detailed description of the children's speech and language skills than previous studies have provided—a study began early after onset and continued longitudinally. Particularly, we advocate the detailed comparison of language skills to other intellectual skills measured nonverbally; of comprehension skills to production skills; and of each to the normal developmental progression. In a later section of this paper, children participating in the pilot study of acquired aphasia carried out at the Waisman Center (1981) will be used to illustrate this approach. Groups homogeneous with respect to the pattern, type, and degree of delay or disorder are far more likely to show similarities in cause, recovery, and effective treatment approaches.

When detailed descriptions of children's cognitive and communication skills are available, a second promising line of new research can then be followed: that of comparing different subsets to discover which share similar problems. We illustrate this second direction for research by comparing three acquired-aphasic and three language-disordered learning-disabled children in a final section of this paper.

Describing Language Skills
of Children with Acquired Aphasia

Over a 24-month period, children suspected of acquired aphasia associated with seizures or abnormal EEGs were seen at an experimental neurogenics clinic at the Waisman Center. The number of visits for each child varied depending upon when during this 24-month period he or she was initially seen. Generally, children were seen for re-evaluation at approximately three-month intervals. The protocol for evaluating language and cognitive functioning in these children was constructed to span a broad developmental range, to include comprehension measures of both vocabulary and syntax, to include production measures of both vocabulary and syntax based on free-speech samples, and to use cognitive measures that were nonverbal in their requirements for both understanding the directions and answering. If children showed very little comprehension on the standard tests, then written testing, or spoken testing with the addition of lip-reading cues, was attempted. Specific procedures included the following:

Standard Assessment Protocol for Pilot Subjects

Comprehension
1. Lexical Comprehension Items (Miller, Chapman, Branston, & Reichle, 1980).
2. Peabody Picture Vocabulary Test (Dunn & Dunn, 1981).
3. Simple Sentence Test Procedure (Chapman & Miller, 1980).
4. Miller-Yoder Test of Grammatical Comprehension (Miller & Yoder, 1972).
5. Revised Token Test (McNeil & Prescott, 1978).
6. Comprehension in Routine Contexts (Miller & Chapman, 1980).

Production Data
1. Conversation with the clinician about current activities and events.
2. Narration—Story-telling about an event, movie, TV show of interest to the child.

Production Analysis
1. Assigning Structural Stage (ASS) (Miller, 1981).
2. MLU/Age Predictions (Miller & Chapman, 1981).
3. Lexical Analysis (Miller & Chapman, 1982).
4. Productivity Analysis (Miller & Chapman, 1982).

Cognitive Assessment

Nonverbal cognitive testing was carried out for each subject whose cognitive abilities had not been previously assessed, using one or more of the following procedures as appropriate:

1. 2—24 months—Piagetian procedures for the sensorimotor period (Miller, Chapman, Branston, & Reichle, 1980).
2. 25—42 months—Leiter International Performance Scale (Leiter, 1969).
3. 42 months—10 years—Columbia Mental Maturity Scale (Burgemeister, Blum & Lorge, 1972).
4. 10 years and up—WISC Performance Scale (Wechsler, 1974).

Procedures appropriate to the child's developmental level were given over one to two continuous days, interspersed with neurological and other behavioral clinical evaluation procedures, including hearing and speech motor control assessment.

Pilot Data

An initial goal of this pilot project was to evaluate similarities and differences in child performance, relative to developmental history and neurological status. After careful examination of cognitive and linguistic data, eight of the sixteen children evaluated fell outside even the most general definition of acquired aphasia in children. Significant cognitive or emotional deficits were uncovered—or a developmental language delay was evident—throughout the developmental period, but no seizure activity was noted.

The remaining eight children could be classed as follows: (1) those whose history of language development could not be clearly established as normal, but who evidenced seizure activity and language deficits affecting both comprehension and production—these were not further classified; (2) children meeting the definition of acquired aphasia who showed no oral language comprehension skills and little productive language, possibly an auditory agnosia group; and (3) children meeting the definition of acquired aphasia whose language comprehension was moderately affected with more severe deficits in language production. It will be helpful to review each group in more detail at this point before moving on to specific comparisons of selected subjects.

Children with Seizures But No History
of Normal Language Development

Three children in the group of eight did not meet the definition of acquired aphasia because no history of normal speech and language development was reported; all, however, displayed a seizure disorder and abnormal EEGs. A brief discussion of each of these children's cognitive, language, and speech performance will help illustrate the point that language disorders—developmental or acquired—can be heterogeneous.

The disorder for one male who was 5 years, 3 months of age was characterized by fluctuation in language and cognitive skills accompanied by repeated episodes of seizures. History indicated that the development of language was generally slow, but he was producing 2- and 3-word utterances by 4 years. During his fourth year, a notable regression in cognitive and language skills was noted in association with seizures. At the time of assessment, cognitive abilities were estimated to be at the 6-month level of functioning (Piagetian sensorimotor stage III). These findings indicate approximately a 57-month difference between his chronological age (63 months) and estimated mental age (6 months). In relation to his cognitive skills, which were estimated to be at the 40-45-month level prior to the seizure disorder, this 57-month difference represents a significant regression in cognitive functioning. Comprehension testing revealed no response to either verbal or nonverbal auditory stimuli. His ability to comprehend language was estimated to be well below the 12-month level of functioning. Expressive speech and language skills were characterized by "grunts" and the production of a few vowel sounds (/a/ and / ə /). No evidence was given that he was attaching meaning to these productions. As was the case with both cognitive and receptive language skills, expressive speech and language abilities were well below the one-year level.

A second child, who was 10 years, 5 months of age, also displayed a language deficit associated with a seizure disorder and abnormal EEG results. For this child, previous reports revealed a long history of language and cognitive delay. However, in contrast to the first child, there was virtually no regression observed in communication and cognitive abilities, even after episodes of seizure activity. Assessment results showed a mild delay in cognitive functioning (based on nonverbal measures). Both lexical and syntactic comprehension were at approximately the 7-year level (CA=10;5). Expressive language was characterized by developmental articulation and syntax errors, and mean length of utterance in morphemes (Brown, 1973) was beyond Stage V. In addition, difficulty in recalling appropriate lexical items was noted during conversational speech.

A third child, 8 years, 4 months of age, also presented a history of general language delay similar to child 1 and child 2. Once again, seizure activity and abnormal EEGs were reported. However, unlike the two previous children, assessment results indicated that nonverbal cognitive abilities were within normal limits. Lexical as well as syntactic comprehension were at the seven-year level of functioning. Expressive language was characterized by both developmental and nondevelopmental syntactic errors. As was the case for child 2, word-finding problems were observed in conversational speech.

Children with Acquired Aphasia, No Comprehension, and Little Production: Auditory Verbal Agnosia?

Two of the children in the pilot study, ages 6 years, 10 months, and 11 years, 8 months, displayed both receptive and expressive language deficits following a normal period of language development. The disturbance in language abilities was associated with seizures and abnormal EEG results. For these children, the language disturbance was characterized by complete loss of auditory comprehension and expressive language abilities, despite retention of age-appropriate cognitive functioning, as measured by nonverbal tasks.

Comprehension data for both children indicated that they were able to discriminate between nonspeech sounds with a high degree of accuracy. As these sounds (environmental sounds and musical instruments) became less familiar, accuracy decreased. Their ability to discriminate between various types of linguistic stimuli was at chance levels. Baseline scores on the Peabody Picture Vocabulary Test could not be obtained when administered with only auditory cues (auditory only = hearing only the spoken lexical item), nor when given using both auditory and visual cues (auditory + visual = hearing the spoken lexical item and seeing the clinician's facial/oral structures). Each child's ability to comprehend language was aided by gestures, signs, and comprehension strategies. Their ability to comprehend spoken language was below the 12-month level of functioning, as indicated by informal comprehension testing. Finally, for the 11-year-old, it is interesting to note that, despite his deficit in auditory comprehension of spoken language, he was capable of correctly matching several orthographically presented words to an appropriate picture. When the PPVT and the Miller-Yoder Test of Grammatical Comprehension were presented orthographically, scores on these measures improved considerably. Due to the 6-year-old's low reading level, comprehension of language could not be tested by orthographic presentation. For both children, auditory comprehension (on the basis of acoustic cues alone) was stable and nonexistent across the 18 to 24 months that they were followed.

On initial evaluation, expressive speech and language for the 11-year-old was characterized by the spontaneous production of several CV, VC, and CVC combinations. Although these productions were mostly unintelligible, he appeared to be attaching meaning to these sound combinations. Production of consonant-vowel combinations, as well as monosyllable words, was enhanced, somewhat, when a model was presented which he could imitate. Based on diagnostic data from this child, it appears that when certain combinations of cues were presented by the clinician (auditory, visual, and orthographic), correct production was enhanced. In addition, during production of isolated phonemes and consonant-vowel combinations, movements of the articulators were apraxic-like. Furthermore, pitch, loudness, and voice quality were not within normal limits. For example, fundamental frequency was extremely high in conversational speech (440 to 460 cycles per second) and there were difficulties in regulating intensity. Voice quality was similar to that of a deaf child. Over the 24-month period this child was followed, little change in expressive speech and language skills were observed.

The 6-year-old, on the other hand, presented virtually no expressive speech and language during the intial assessment. However, for this child, gains in productive speech were documented across the 18 months she was followed. At first, imitation of sounds and words, or spontaneous production of vowels were observed. During later evaluations, expressive speech and language consisted of several 1- and 2-word utterances with good intelligibility.

Three distinguishing characteristics of these two children include (1) a disturbance in normal language development, (2) presence of seizures and abnormal EEG findings, and (3) the retention of normal nonverbal cognitive functions. A fourth, and possibly the most interesting aspect, of the disorder in these children is related to their unique comprehension abilities. That is, regardless of their ability to discriminate between certain nonlinguistic auditory stimuli, they, in essence, display verbal auditory agnosia (pure word deafness). As noted by Rapin et al. (1977) and Campbell and Heaton (1979), among others, sight-word-reading vocabulary is typically in advance of such children's auditory receptive language skills. In some, visual communication functions are remarkably preserved, and many can be taught to read and write quite well. Higher levels of comprehension abilities assessed through other channels in these children are striking, especially when they are compared to congenitally hearing-impaired children learning oral and written language. Comprehension skills in this latter group for written language are greatly delayed. Assuming that the two children described above might have begun learning language over again through lip reading, sign, and written programming after the onset of the convulsive disorder, they came much further in comprehension than one could reasonably expect under the circumstances.

Thus, these two children, along with similar cases described in the literature, indicate that the language loss at the time of the seizure episodes was not irrevocable. Rather, these case descriptions suggest that the links between acoustic input and meaning, and between meaning and expression, were severed—double dissociation, in the aphasiologist's terms. If this hypothesis is so, one should be able to demonstrate extraordinarily rapid acquisition of language through an augmentative system (e.g., signing and writing) that maps directly into previously acquired linguistic knowledge. Furthermore, one could predict that expression in such an augmentative system would be representative of language organization prior to the disorder. Neither of these hypotheses is true for congenitally hearing-impaired children, nor should they prove true if the seizure disorder, in fact, "erased" prior language learning. At present, the disturbance in linguistic competence (as opposed to language performance measured through verbal language comprehension and production) in these children is poorly understood and, thus, is a good candidate for further inquiry. The study of these childrens' language learning and knowledge, through augmentative procedures, may provide important pieces of information to this puzzling question.

Children with Acquired Aphasia, Variable Comprehension, and Delayed Production with Word Finding Problems

The last three children in the pilot study showed auditory comprehension and expressive speech and language abilities which appear to be both quantitatively and qualitatively different from those previously described. These three children (ages 9, 10, and 11 years) also experienced a normal period of speech and language development. Between ages 4 and 7 years, disturbances in receptive and expressive language skills were observed, accompanied by a seizure disorder. The disturbances in communication abilities proved to be less severe than the loss displayed by the children presented previously. When improvement in speech and language took place, it was sudden. Psychological and school reports indicated that nonverbal cognitive abilities were not affected and the major educational deficits occurred in academic areas, such as spelling and reading. Our clinical observations of these three children indicate that, although they are capable of functioning in a normal educational setting, they continue to display specific receptive and expressive language deficits which interfere with the normal learning process. Expressive speech and language is characterized by developmental and nondevelopmental syntactic errors, word finding problems, and other communication breakdowns. Aside from developmental articulation errors, speech is relatively intelligible. In terms of receptive language, variable auditory comprehension of the same word or strings of words has been observed from moment to moment. In addition, all three of these children claim that they have increased difficulty processing spontaneous speech when it is produced at rates they perceive as being faster than normal.

The description of the abilities of these three children is continued in the following section, where we compare their productive language to learning-disabled language-disordered children with no history of seizures or sudden disturbance of language functioning.

Comparing the Expressive Language of Aphasic and Learning Disabled Children

Do children with acquired aphasia associated with a seizure disorder show productive language similar to children with language deficits accompanied by learning disabilities? Descriptive and causal models attempting to explain the performance of language-delayed learning-disabled children have been primarily unidimensional, and presented as hypotheses about the impaired processes. These hypotheses include deficits in:

1. Short-term memory
2. Rate of auditory processing
3. Auditory sequencing
4. Linguistic processing
5. Phonological processing
6. Attention
7. Production-span capacity
8. Rhythmic ability
9. Hierarchical planning
10. General representation

It can be argued that all of these conditions simply co-occur with delayed onset and slow rates of language acquisition. Or, one could argue they are the result, rather than the cause, of the language disorder. At present there are no direct prognostic links from deficits in any specific process or physiological condition to the course, sequence, rate, and extent of language and communication development; but, children have not been grouped by detailed patterns of language deficit prior to the investigation of these factors, and comprehension status, in particular, has seldom been documented.

Each of the hypotheses proposed above predicts certain outcomes for language comprehension and language production independently; and each hypothesis could be extended, if warranted by similarities in functioning, to children with acquired aphasia. Short-term memory deficits, slow rate of auditory processing, deficits in linguistic and phonological processing, and attentional deficits would result in a disturbance in language comprehension. Reduced production-span capacity would directly affect language production at a variety of levels. Sequencing deficits, defective rhythmic abilities, hierarchical planning deficits, and general representational deficits would impair both language comprehension and production. When detailed language-performance data become available on children within each of the two groups, it may be possible to predict processing deficits with sufficient specificity to test them experimentally. Here, we illustrate one fragment of the comparison in language skills necessary to warrant the hypothesis that similar processing problems may be at work for the two different groups.

In order to examine the question of whether acquired aphasic and language disordered children showed similar deficits in talking, analyses of productive language were carried out using a computer program entitled Systematic Analysis of Language Transcripts (SALT) (Miller & Chapman, 1982). This program permits transcripts to be typed in, stored, and analyzed for both adults and children for the following measures: mean length of utterance in words and morphemes; distribution of utterances by word and morpheme length; distribution of number of utterances per speaking turn; total number of words; total number of different words; type-token ratio; frequency of occurrence of each word in the sample; bound morpheme frequency table; question, negation, conjunction, modal verb, semi-auxiliary frequency tables; and a search routine to recall utterances containing specific words, word sets, or word strings. The latter can be used to analyze subjects' use of vocabulary containing various semantic fields, such as time words, mental verbs, and words making indefinite reference.

Aphasic Children

The aphasic children selected for comparison were three boys, ages 9;10, 10;0, and 11;6, who fell into the third group described previously. These children had experienced a normal period of speech and language development. Between the ages of 4 and 7 years, a disturbance in auditory comprehension and expressive language skills was noted, accompanied by a seizure disorder and abnormal EEGs, which were characterized by a left temporal lobe focus. At the time of testing, all children displayed normal nonverbal cognitive abilities, and were attending a normal educational classroom. Descriptive data consisting of age, sex, developmental history, time of onset, seizure history, EEG findings, educational history, and cognitive, comprehension, and productions levels are summarized in Table 3-4.

Learning-Disabled Children

The language-delayed learning-disabled children selected for comparison with the aphasic children were two boys and one girl, ages 11;2, 11;3, and 10;11, who had been identified as learning-disabled by the public schools. Medical history revealed that none of these children had displayed seizures or other neurological abnormalities. At the time of testing, all showed a 28 to 36 point gap between verbal and performance scale IQ scores on the Wechsler Intelligence Scale for Children (Revised), with performance scale scores being the higher of the two. All were attending a class for children with specific learning disabilities. Descriptive data for these children are summarized in Table 3-5.

Language Samples

Spontaneous language samples were obtained under two conditions: (1) a conversational condition in which the child engaged in dialogue concerning past, present, and future events, and (2) a narrative condition in which the child described a television show from memory. Conversational and narrative language samples from acquired aphasic and LD (learning-disabled) children were analyzed for a variety of lexical and productive characteristics.

Mean Length of Utterance

Tables 3-6 and 3-7 present word and morpheme summaries for conversation and narration conditions for both aphasic and LD children. With regard to utterance length for complete and intelligible utterances, mean length of utterance (MLU) in morphemes (Brown, 1973) for the conversational condition ranged from 4.22 to 5.86 for the aphasic children, and from 4.73 to 5.47 for the LD children. During the narrative condition, MLU ranged from 4.67 to 8.10 for the aphasic group, and from 5.43 to 8.69 for the LD children. As these data indicate, similar ranges for MLU were obtained for aphasic and LD groups, for both conditions. However, with the exception of LD6, each aphasic and LD child presented a greater MLU for narration than conversation.

Table 3-4.
Descriptive characteristics of the aphasic children.

Category	Children		
	AP1	*AP2*	*AP3*
Age	9;10	11;6	10;0
Sex	Male	Male	Male
Developmental History	Normal until age 4;0 when seizures began.	Normal until age 5;6 when seizures began.	Mild early expressive language delay; first word at 18 months; 2-word utterances at 42 months.
Time of Onset of Language Disturbance	4;0	5;0-7;0	5;0
Seizure History	Several petite mal and motor seizures - Abnormal EEG— Predominately left temporal region.	Several motor seizures at night— Abnormal EEG— left temporal region.	Several motor seizures at night— Abnormal EEG— left temporal region

Educational History	Attended a special school for aphasic children from 4;0 to 7;0—Currently in a normal 4th grade class.	Has always been in a normal educational classroom setting.	Has always been in a normal classroom setting.
Cognition	80%-ile— Ravens Matrices	60%-ile— Ravens Matrices	WISC-R V 90 P 118 FS 104
Comprehension	PPVT—6;2 Miller-Yoder— 100%.	PPVT—9;2 Miller-Yoder— 100%.	PPVT—6;5 Miller-Yoder— 100%.
Production	MLU 5.10 Word retrieval problems.	MLU 5.86 Word retrieval problems.	MLU 4.22 Word retrieval problems.

Table 3-5
Descriptive characteristics of the learning-disabled children. (NA = not available)

Category	Children		
	LD1	*LD2*	*LD3*
Age	11;2	11;3	10;11
Sex	Male	Male	Female
Developmental History	Normal	Normal	Normal
Time of Onset of Language Disturbance.	N/A	N/A	N/A
Seizure History	N/A	N/A	N/A
Educational History	Has been in both normal and LD classroom—currently in a LD classroom.	Has been in normal and LD classrooms—currently in LD classroom.	Has been in both normal and LD classrooms—currently in LD classroom.
Cognition	WISC-R V 98 P 121 FS 104	WISC-R V 95 P 123 FS 108	WISC-R V 81 P 117 FS 97
Comprehension	PPVT—11;0 Miller-Yoder—100%.	PPVT 10;5 Miller-Yoder—100%.	PPVT 9;10 Miller-Yoder—100%.
Production	MLU 5.77 Word retrieval problems.	MLU 5.31 Word retrieval problems.	MLU 6.05 Word retrieval problems.

Utterance Types

Tables 3-8 and 3-9 summarize frequency and percentage of utterance types for both groups of children. As can be seen in these two tables, percentage of complete and intelligible utterances in the conversational condition was high, ranging from 88.89% to 96.61% for the aphasic group, and from 96.26% to 100.00% for the LD group. In the narrative condition, percentage of complete and intelligible utterances ranged from 83.75% to 96.67% for the three aphasic children, and from 78.16% to 98.88% for the three LD children. As shown, the percentage of complete and intelligible utterances is similar for each group, for both conversational and narrative conditions. However, for the majority of children, the percentage of complete and intelligible utterances decreases slightly in the narrative condition.

Communication Breakdowns

Conversational and narrative samples were also analyzed in terms of communication breakdowns, defined as including:

1. Garbles, which involve:
   a. filled pauses
   b. part-word repetitions
   c. whole-word repetitions
   d. phrase repetitions
   e. word/phrase replacements
   f. word/phrase revisions;
2. Incomplete utterances (abandoned utterance attempts); and
3. Unintelligible or partially unintelligible utterances;

Table 3-10 provides a summary of the overall percentage of communication breakdowns for each child per-language-sample-condition (i.e., conversation vs. narration). Based on this summary information, several points can be made. First, it is evident that for both groups, the percentage of communication breakdowns was higher for the narrative sample than for the conversational sample. It is possible to speculate that the higher percentage of communication breakdowns in the narrative condition was due to increased processing demands involved in reconstructing and reorganizing information from memory. Alternately, it could be reasoned that communication breakdowns occurred more frequently during the narrative sample as a result of attempts to produce longer and more syntactically complex utterances. The data in Table 3-11 seem to support the latter interpretation. As previously noted, MLU for complete and intelligible utterances in the narrative sample (for all subjects except LD6) was higher

132268

Table 3-6
Aphasic children word and morpheme summaries.

	Conversation								
	Child AP1 Con		Child AP2 Con		Child AP3 Con	
	Total Utterances	Complete and Intelligible	Total Utterances	Complete and Intelligible	Total Utterances	Complete and Intelligible
No. Different Words	183	174	135	129	153	142
Total No. Words	534	490	341	307	360	305
TTR (First 50 utterances)	---	0.50	---	0.45	---	0.54
MLU in Words	4.64	4.58	5.33	5.39	3.75	3.81
MLU in Morphemes	5.15	5.10	5.83	5.86	4.12	4.22
Brown's Stage	Post V	Post V	Post V	Post V	Late V	Late V

Narration

	Child AP1 Nar		Child AP2 Nar		Child AP3 Nar	
	Total Utterances	Complete and Intelligible	Total Utterances	Complete and Intelligible	Total Utterances	Complete and Intelligible
No. Different Words	143	126	178	160	126	116
Total No. Words	375	302	619	479	274	237
TTR (First 50 utterances)	---	0.42	---	0.40	---	0.50
MLU in Words	6.15	6.29	6.96	7.15	4.09	4.09
MLU in Morphemes	6.84	6.98	7.85	8.10	4.63	4.67
Brown's Stage	Post V	Post V	Post V	Post V	Post V	Post V

Table 3-7.
Learning-Disabled children word and morpheme summaries.

| | Conversation | | | | | |
| | Child LD1 Con | | Child LD2 Con | | Child LD3 Con | |
	Total Utterances	Complete and Intelligible	Total Utterances	Complete and Intelligible	Total Utterances	Complete and Intelligible
No. Different Words	221	221	165	164	329	320
Total No. Words	662	657	456	454	1060	985
TTR (First 50 utterances)	---	0.53	---	0.49	---	0.51
MLU in Words	4.98	5.05	4.65	4.73	5.52	5.47
MLU in Morphemes	5.68	5.77	5.22	5.31	6.09	6.05
Brown's Stage	Post V	Post V	Post V	Post V	Post V	Post V

Narration

	Child LD1 Nar		Child LD2 Nar		Child LD3 Nar	
	Total Utterances	Complete and Intelligible	Total Utterances	Complete and Intelligible	Total Utterances	Complete and Intelligible
No. Different Words	205	202	136	133	196	170
Total No. Words	706	693	371	349	472	335
TTR (First 50 utterances)	---	0.40	---	0.38	---	0.55
MLU in Words	7.84	7.87	6.87	7.12	5.36	4.93
MLU in Morphemes	8.66	8.69	7.44	7.71	5.85	5.43
Brown's Stage	Post V	Post V	Post V	Post V	Post V	Post V

Table 3-8
Aphasic children frequency and percentage of utterance types.

	Conversation								
	Child AP1 Con		Child AP2 Con			Child AP3 Con		
	Number	%	Number	%		Number	%	
Total Utterances (Speaker Attempts)	115	---	64	---		97	---	
(Utterances with Garbles)	36	31.30	12	18.75		27	27.84	
Complete Utterances	112	97.39	59	92.19		90	92.78	
Unintelligible	0	---	0	---		4	4.44	
Partly intelligible	5	4.46	2	3.39		6	6.67	
Complete and intelligible	107	95.54	57	96.61		80	88.89	
Incomplete Utterances	3	2.61	5	7.81		6	6.19	
Unintelligible	0	---	0	---		0	---	
Partly intelligible	0	---	1	20.00		0	---	
Incomplete and intelligible	3	100.00	4	80.00		6	100.00	

Narration

	Child AP1 Nar		Child AP2 Nar		Child AP3 Nar	
	Number	%	Number	%	Number	%
Total Utterances (Speaker Attempts)	61	---	89	---	67	---
(Utterances with Garbles)	26	42.62	31	34.83	26	38.81
Complete Utterances	54	88.52	80	89.89	60	89.55
Unintelligible	0	---	0	---	0	---
Partly intelligible	6	11.11	13	16.25	2	3.33
Complete and intelligible	48	88.89	67	83.75	58	96.67
Incomplete Utterances	7	11.48	9	10.11	7	10.45
Unintelligible	0	---	1	11.11	0	---
Partly intelligible	0	---	0	---	1	14.29
Incomplete and intelligible	7	100.00	8	88.89	6	85.71

Table 3-9
Learning-disabled children frequency and percentage of utterance types.

	Conversation					
	Child LD1 Con		Child LD2 Con		Child LD3 Con	
	Number	%	Number	%	Number	%
Total Utterances (Speaker Attempts)	133	---	98	---	192	---
(Utterances with Garbles)	25	18.88	27	27.55	42	21.87
Complete Utterances	**130**	**97.74**	**96**	**97.96**	**187**	**97.40**
Unintelligible	0	---	0	---	1	0.53
Partly intelligible	0	---	0	---	6	3.21
Complete and intelligible	130	100.00	96	100.00	180	96.26
Incomplete Utterances	**3**	**2.26**	**2**	**2.04**	**5**	**2.60**
Unintelligible	0	---	0	---	0	---
Partly intelligible	0	---	0	---	0	---
Incomplete and intelligible	3	100.00	2	100.00	5	100.00

Narration

	Child LD1 Nar		Child LD2 Nar		Child LD3 Nar	
	Number	*%*	*Number*	*%*	*Number*	*%*
Total Utterances (Speaker Attempts)	91	---	55	---	90	---
(Utterances with Garbles)	26	28.57	25	45.45	44	48.89
Complete Utterances	89	97.80	50	90.91	87	96.67
Unintelligible	0	---	0	---	4	4.60
Partly intelligible	1	1.12	1	2.00	15	17.24
Complete and intelligible	88	98.88	49	98.00	68	78.16
Incomplete Utterances	1	1.10	4	7.27	1	1.11
Unintelligible	0	---	0	---	0	---
Partly intelligible	0	---	0	---	0	---
Incomplete and intelligible	1	100.00	4	100.00	1	100.00
Communication Gesture	1	1.10	1	1.82	2	2.22

Table 3-10
Percentage of utterances containing communication breakdowns
by sample condition.

Children	Conversation	Narrative
AP1	32	54
AP2	30	56
AP3	34	46
LD1	21	28
LD2	26	47
LD3	25	56

than MLU for complete and intelligible utterances in the conversational sample. Furthermore, within each language sample condition, the MLU for the utterances containing garbles is higher in every case than the MLU for the entire sample. That is, utterances in which filled pauses, part-word repetitions, etc., occurred were generally longer than those without these types of commmunication breakdowns. Words and phrases within garbles were, of course, excluded from the MLU count—only the remainder of the utterance was counted.

Also evident in Table 3-10 is the fact that the acquired aphasic group had somewhat higher percentages of communication breakdowns for the conversational condition (ranging from 30-34%) than the LD group (ranging from 21-26%). However, two of the three LD children (LD3 and LD6) evidenced percentages of breakdowns in the narrative conditions which were nearly identical to those of the aphasic children. The third LD child (LD2) demonstrated relatively low percentages of communication breakdowns across both sample conditions.

Data on the various categories of communication breakdowns for the acquired aphasic children and the LD children are presented in Tables 3-12 and 3-13, respectively. In Table 3-14, these data are summarized in terms of mean percentages exhibited by both groups for each breakdown category in the conversational condition and the narrative condition. The results of these analyses point to several similarities between the two groups. It is evident that the finding regarding higher percentages of communication breakdowns on the narrative samples than the conversational samples also generally hold true for the individual categories of breakdowns. More importantly, the pattern of types of communication breakdowns that occur most frequently were very similar across groups. Regardless of language-sample condition (conversational vs. narrative), the breakdown types most common in aphasic and LD children were filled pauses and word/phrase revisions. Filled pauses in the transcripts of the aphasic children consisted exclusively of fillers "um" or "uh", as in "well (um) when (um um) we play tag," while interjections such as "and my sister is (oh boy is tw) twelve" were used by the LD children in addition to fillers. Word revisions, such as in the utterance "go to my (cousin) cousin's house," usually involved the addition of a grammatical marker to the unmarked form. Phrase revisions, for example "in fourth grade (um I was like, I came, I came like) I was asleep" entailed syntactic reformations at the phrase level.

Communication breakdowns exhibited by the acquired aphasic children and the LD children appear to be related, at least in some instances, to word-retrieval difficulties. There were varying degrees of evidence in the transcripts indicative of word-finding problems. Some of the most obvious, but infrequent, cases involved repairs, or instances in which the child eventually recalled the appropriate word, as illustrated by the following example: "It's only hard to because they always put these (uh, a lot of, uh, hum) *things* on it, (uh) *words*. A lotta *words* on it." There were 10 instances of these types of repairs in the aphasic transcripts (based on a total of 509 utterances) and 6 instances (in 659 total utterances) in the LD transcripts. Direct remarks such as "oh, what is it called" or "starts with a Y" also provided clear indications of word-finding problems. Such comments, however, were rare. Other evidence of difficulties in word retrieval included the use of semantically or phonologically related words for the intended word, such as the use of "remind" for "remember," or "where" for "when". There were 10 instances of semantically similar word replacement in the transcripts of the aphasic children and only 1 instance in the transcripts of the LD children. Phonological replacements occurred 3 times in the aphasic samples and once in the LD samples. A less direct form of evidence for word-retrieval problems involved the use of indefinite reference terms where definite reference was called for, including deictic terms with no clear referent, and nonspecific terms such as "stuff" and "things." In the aphasic transcripts, indefinite reference terms appeared 46 times as compared to 31 times in the LD transcripts (which is a difference of 9% compared to 5% of the total utterances).

Whether word-finding problems can eventually be shown to be the root of the other communication breakdowns observed, or not, the overall comparison of language use in the two groups reveals striking similarities. Naive listeners could not distinguish among brief segments of narration from

Table 3-11
Mean utterance length in morphemes of total samples and the utterances containing garbles by child.

	Conversational Sample		Narrative Sample	
Child	Total Sample	Utterances with Garbles	Total Sample	Utterances with Garbles
AP1	5.10	6.90	6.98	10.15
AP2	5.86	9.42	8.10	10.92
AP3	4.22	6.05	4.67	5.70
LD1	5.77	7.20	8.69	13.52
LD2	5.31	8.67	7.71	10.2
LD3	6.05	8.70	5.43	7.79

Table 3-12
Percentage of aphasic children's total utterances containing each type of communication breakdown.

Child/ Sample	Filled Pauses	Part-word Repetition	Whole-word Repetition	Phrase Repetition	Word/Phrase Replacement	Word/Phrase Revision	Incomplete Utterance	Unintelligible Utterance
AP1 CON	11	1	7	7	4	10	3	4
AP1 NAR	21	0	12	10	7	18	12	10
AP2 CON	6	2	9	2	2	9	8	5
AP2 NAR	23	1	15	5	6	9	10	16
AP3 CON	12	3	4	4	0	12	5	9
AP3 NAR	15	3	6	12	0	15	10	5

Table 3-13
Percentage of learning-disordered children's total utterances containing each type of communication breakdown.

Child/ Sample	Filled Pauses	Part-word Repetition	Whole-word Repetition	Phrase Repetition	Word/Phrase Replacement	Word/Phrase Revision	Incomplete Utterance	Unintelligible Utterance
LD1 CON	8	2	2	3	2	5	2	0
LD1 NAR	13	2	2	2	4	8	1	1
LD2 CON	7	2	7	5	2	10	2	0
LD2 NAR	24	2	7	5	5	24	7	2
LD3 CON	10	3	4	2	2	6	3	4
LD3 NAR	23	2	10	3	7	10	1	21

Table 3-14
Mean percentage of total utterances containing each type of communication breakdown by sample condition for acquired aphasic and learning-disabled children.

Children and Sample	Filled Pauses	Part-word Repetition	Whole-word Repetition	Phrase Repetition	Word/Phrase Replacement	Word/Phrase Revision	Incomplete Utterance	Unintelligible Utterance
Aphasic Conversation	10	2	7	4	2	10	5	6
Aphasic Narration	20	1	11	9	4	14	11	10
LD Conversation	8	2	4	3	2	7	2	1
LD Narration	20	2	10	3	5	14	3	8

children in each of the groups. This comparison suggests that similar processes may be at work for the two groups studied: the acquired aphasic children, with only moderate delays in comprehension and production skills, and the learning-disabled children with specific language deficits.

Summary

We have reviewed the work on children with acquired aphasia associated with a seizure disorder, and concluded that detailed descriptions of communication functioning may improve our ability to predict the course of the disorder, monitor the child's improvement, or select appropriate intervention techniques for the child's current status. New directions for research were illustrated through detailed descriptions of communicative functioning in eight children, documenting the potential divergence in linguistic comprehension skills among children, and—through a comparison of a subgroup of acquired aphasic children with language-delayed learning-disabled children of a similar age and linguistic level—documenting the similarities in production characteristics of the two groups. We believe that the research strategy of creating homogeneous groups through detailed description, and comparing homogeneous subsets of language-disordered children will improve the clinician's ability to predict the course of recovery and make recommendations for treatment.

Acknowledgments

Support for this project came in part from research grants to the first author from the Graduate School Research Committee, University of Wisconsin-Madison, MRRC core support to the first and third authors through the Waisman Center on Mental Retardation and Human Development, University of Wisconsin-Madison, NICHD, NIH, Grant No. 2-P30-HD-03352-14, and support from University Affiliated Facility Project No. MCT-000915-13 to the Waisman Center. Portions of this work were conducted as part of a clinical research project coordinated by Dr. Kurt Hecox.

References

Barlow, C.F. Acquired disorders of communication in childhood. In A. Dorfman, (Ed.), *Child care in health and disease.* Chicago: Year Book Medical, 1968.

Brown, R. *A first language.* Cambridge, MA: Harvard University Press, 1973.

Burgemeister, B., Blum, L., & Lorge, I. *Columbia Mental Maturity Scale* (3rd Ed.). N.Y.: Harcourt, Brace & Jovanovich, 1972.

Campbell, T.F. *Effects of presentation rate and divided attention on auditory comprehension in acquired childhood aphasia.* Unpublished doctoral dissertation, University of Wisconsin, 1982.

Campbell, T.F. & Heaton, E.M. An expressive speech program for a child with acquired aphasia: A case study. *Canadian Journal of Human Communication,* 1978, Summer, 89-102.

Campbell, T.F., & Heaton, E.M. An expressive language program for a child with acquired aphasia. Paper presented at the Annual Convention of the American Speech-Language-Hearing Association, Atlanta, 1979.

Chapman, R., & Miller, J. *The simple sentence comprehension procedure.* Unpublished paper, University of Wisconsin-Madison, 1980.

Cooper, J.A., & Ferry, P.C. Acquired auditory verbal aphasia and seizures in childhood. *Journal of Speech and Hearing Disorders,* 1978, *43,* 176-184.

Cromer, R. Hierarchical ordering disability and aphasic children. In P. Dale & D. Ingram (Eds.), *Child language—An international perspective.* Baltimore: University Park Press, 1981, pp. 319-330.

de Negri, M. Some critical notes about "the epilepsy-aphasia syndrome" in children. *Brain Development,* 1980, *2,* 81-85.

Deonna, T.H. Beaumanoir, F., Gaillard, F., & Assal, G. Acquired aphasia in childhood with seizure disorder: A heterogeneous syndrome. *Neuropadiatrie,* 1977, *8,* 3, 263-273.

Deonna, T., Fletcher, P., & Voumard, C. Temporary regression during language acquisition: A linguistic analysis of a 2½ year old child with epileptic aphasia. *Developmental Medicine and Child Neurology,* in press.

Deuel, R.K., & Lenn, N.J. Acquired epileptic aphasia. Paper presented at the Child Neurology Society Meeting, Madison, WI, 1974.

Deuel, R.K., & Lenn, N.J. Treatment of acquired epileptic aphasia. *Journal of Pediatrics,* 1977, *90,* 959-961.

Dunn, L.M., & Dunn, L.M. *Peabody Picture Vocabulary Test-Revised.* Circle Pines, MI: American Guidance Service, 1981.

Gascon, G., Victor, O. Lombroso, C.T., & Goodglass, H. Language disorder, convulsive disorder and electroencephalographic abnormalities. *Archives of Neurology,* 1973, *28,* 156-162.

Harel, S.H., Walsh, G.O., & Menkes, J.H. Syndrome of acquired aphasia with epileptic electroencephalographic discharges. Paper presented at the Child Neurology Society Meeting, Nashville, Tenn., 1973.

Holmes, G.L., & McKeever, M. Aphasia with EEG abnormalities: Evaluation using EEG telemetry and videotape recording. *Neurology,* 1981, *31,* 102.

Huskisson, J.A. Acquired receptive language difficulties in childhood: A case study. *British Journal of Disorders of Communication,* 1974, *8,* 54-63.

Johnston, J. The language disordered child. In N. Lass, L. McReynolds, J. Northern, & D. Yoder (Eds.), *Speech, language and hearing: Vol. II. Pathologies of speech and language.* Philadelphia: W.B. Sanders, 1982, 780-801.

Jordan, L.S. Receptive and expressive language problems occurring in combination with a seizure disorder: A case report. *Journal of Communication Disorders,* 1980, *13,* 295-303.

Koepp, P., & Lagenstein I. Acquired epileptic aphasia: Letter to the editor. *The Journal of Pediatrics,* 1978, *99,* 164.

Kracke, I. Perception of rhythmic sequences by receptive aphasic and deaf children. *British Journal of Disorders of Communication,* 1978, *13,* 43-51.

Landau, W.M., & Kleffner, F.R. Syndrome of acquired aphasia with convulsive disorder in children. *Neurology,* 1957, *10,* 915-921.

Leiter, R.G. *Leiter International Performance Scale.* Los Angeles: Western Psychological Services, 1969.

Leonard, L. Language impairment in children. *Merrill-Palmer Quarterly,* 1979, *25,* 205-232.

Lou, H.C., Brandt, S., & Bruhn, P. Progressive aphasia and epilepsy with a self-limited course. In J.K. Penry (Ed.), *Epilepsy: The eighth international symposium.* New York: Raven Press (1977).

Mantovani, J.F., & Landau, W.M. Acquired aphasics with convulsive disorder: Course and prognosis. *Neurology,* 1980, *30,* 524-529.

McKinney, W., & McGreal, D.A. An asphasic syndrome in children. *Canadian Medical Association Journal,* 1974, *110,* 637-639.

McNeil, M.R., & Prescott, T.E. *Revised Token Test.* Baltimore: University Park Press, 1978.

Miller, J. *Assessing language production in children.* Baltimore: University Park Press, 1981.

Miller, J., & Chapman, R. Comprehension in routine contexts, Unpublished paper, University of Wisconsin-Madison, 1980.

Miller, J., & Chapman, R. The relationship between age and mean length of utterance in morphemes. *Journal of Speech and Hearing Research,* 1981, *24,* 154-161.

Miller, J., & Chapman, R. Users Manual: (SALT) Systematic Analysis of Language Transcripts. Unpublished document, University of Wisconsin-Madison, 1982.

Miller, J.F., Chapman, R., Branston, MB. & Reichle, J. Language comprehension in sensorimotor stages V and VI. *Journal of Speech and Hearing Research,* 1980, *23,* 284-311.

Miller, J.F., & Yoder, D.E. *The Miller-Yoder Test of Grammatical Comprehension.* Madison, WS: The University Book Store, 1972.

Rapin, I., Mattis, S., Rowan, A.J., & Golden, G.G. Verbal auditory agnosia in children. *Developmental Medicine and Child Neurology,* 1977, *19,* 192-207.

Rasmussen, T., & McCann, W. Clinical studies of patients with focal epilepsy due to chronic encephalitis. *Transactions of the American Neurological Association,* 1968, *93,* 89-94.

Rose, F.C. Receptive aphasia in childhood. Proceedings of the Society of British Neurological Surgeons. *Journal of Neurology, Neurosurgery and Psychiatry,* 1969, *32,* 65. (Abstract)

Sato, S., & Dreifuss, F.E. Electroencephalographic findings in a patient with developmental expressive aphasia. *Neurology,* 1972, *23,* 181-185.

Shoumaker, R.D., Bennett, D.R., Bray, P.F. & Curless, R.G. Clinical and EEG manifestations of an unusual aphasic syndrome in children. *Neurology,* 1974, *24,* 10-16.

Stein, L.K., & Curry, E.K.W. Childhood auditory agnosia. *Journal of Speech and Hearing Disorders,* 1968, *28,* 361-370.

Van Harskamp, F., Van Dongen, H.R., & Loonen, M.C.B. Acquired aphasia with convulsive disorders in children: Case study with seven years follow-up. *Brain and Language,* 1978, *6,* 141-148.

Waisman Study. Experimental neurosensory language disorders clinic. Waisman Center of Mental Retardation, University of Wisconsin-Madison, 1981.

Waters, G.V. The syndrome of acquired aphasia and convulsive disorder in children. *Journal of the Canadian Medical Association,* 1974, *110,* 611-612.

Wechsler, D. *Wechsler Intelligence Scale for Children (WISC).* New York: Psychological Corporation, 1974.

Worster-Drought, C. An unusual form of acquired aphasia in children. *Developmental Medicine and Child Neurology,* 1971, *13,* 563-571.

M. Jeanne Wilcox

Developmental Language Disorders: Preschoolers

The current emphasis on pragmatic aspects of communication has resulted in an investigative trend that has important implications for the structure and content of early language intervention. Specifically, studies of child language acquisition have been broadened to include an examination of communicative, rather than purely linguistic, competence. Many early investigations of child language, being largelyinfluenced by Chomsky's works (1957, 1965) focused primarily on the acquisition of linguistic competence (Braine, 1963; Brown, Cazden, & Bellugi, 1973; Brown & Hanlon, 1970; McNeill, 1970). The influence of such investigations has been manifested in a variety of syntactically based early language intervention protocols (e.g., Miller & Yoder, 1972; Stremel & Waryas, 1974). More recently, as a pragmatic view of communication has taken hold, specialists concerned with normal, as well as disordered, child language have realized that linguistic competence is only one portion of the process of language acquisition (Bates, 1976; Hymes, 1971; Lakoff, 1972; Rees, 1978). The focus in studies of child language has therefore shifted from linguistic to communicative competence. As a result of this shift, it has become generally accepted that linguistic structures cannot be studied in normal populations, or treated in disordered populations, without reference to the context in which communication naturally occurs.

The general purpose of this chapter is threefold. First, a brief review of clinically applicable findings pertaining to the acquisition of communicative

© College-Hill Press, Inc. All rights, including that of translation, reserved. No part of this publication may be reproduced without the written permission of the publisher.

competence will be conducted. Second, the integration of these findings into current research focusing on language-disordered preschoolers will be considered. Finally, a treatment model for preschool language intervention will be presented in detail. The model, which is based upon current findings in the normal literature, serves as an example of the application of normal developmental literature to the treatment of language-disordered children.

The Acquisition of Communicative Competence: Implications for Language-Disordered Children

Communicative competence can generally be regarded as the ability to convey effectively and efficiently an intended message to a receiver. As such, this ability requires not only knowledge of the conventional communicative code, but also knowledge pertaining to socially appropriate communicative behaviors. As researchers have attempted to describe the acquisition of communicative competence, several areas have received attention. These include communication prior to speech, analyses of the contexts and functions of communication, the role of environmental communicative input, and children's observance of socially appropriate communicative conventions. Investigation in each of these areas has yielded a wealth of information that merits consideration in the management of young language-disordered children.

Prespeech Communication

Whereas language development was once viewed as beginning with the first word, it has become increasingly clearer that, prior to actual word production, children have developed rich communicative systems. Various researchers have examined children's prespeech communicative abilities (Barten, 1979; Bates, Camaioni, & Volterra, 1979; Bruner, 1975; Carter, 1978; Clark, 1978). It appears that there is a phase of development in which children intentionally communicate without actually using words. Generally, these communications seem to occur by means of gestures which may or may not be accompanied by vocalizations. Several investigators have systematically observed and described such gestural systems (Bates et al., 1979; Carter, 1978; Halliday, 1975).

Results of investigations, such as those cited above, have implied that there is a continuous flow of development from early gestural systems to speech. However, the specific transition from gestural communication to speech has not been specified. Nor is it clear the degree to which early gestures, per se , are required for later speech development. Most children communicate with gestures prior to words. However, when early words emerge, they do not simply replace gestures (Wilcox & Howse, 1982). On the contrary, early words are most often expressed as accompaniments to gestures (Snow, 1981). Further, as verbal development progresses, many gestures increase in frequency (Wilkinson & Rembold, 1981). Thus, prespeech gestural systems do not seem to serve as mere symbols to be later replaced by verbal behavior. Such gestures would seem to play a broader role in the acquisition of communicative competence.

The issue thus becomes one of identifying the role of prespeech communication in overall communicative development. This issue has been addressed by various researchers (Bruner, 1979; Dore, 1974; Halliday, 1975). The bulk of the research suggests that while children are engaging in prespeech communication, they are acquiring important sociocommunicative information. In this way, children who are not yet capable of verbal representation are using gestures as devices for extracting and putting into use knowledge about the communicative process.

The specification of knowledge gained during prespeech communication is particularly important for professionals concerned with programming for the nonverbal language-disordered child. It would seem that prior to the commencement of a verbal intervention plan, it is necessary to ascertain a child's understanding of the communicative concepts that are normally established during prespeech communciation.

For the clinician, the issue becomes one of being able to define operationally the type of communicative knowledge gained during prespeech communication. More specifically, what must a child understand about communication before she or he can engage in effective verbal interactions? The answer to this question seems to lie in the studies of children's language that have focused on early communicative functions.

Social Communicative Functions

Analyses of children's prespeech as well as early verbal communications have indicated that young children are capable of expressing a variety of social language functions, Halliday (1975) has described in detail the emergence of a social language system. Although many other investigators have observed and described prespeech and early verbal communications (e.g., Bates et al., 1979; Carter, 1978; Dore, 1974), Halliday's account relates most directly to the exemplary treatment model to be discussed later in this chapter and will, therefore, be the only description considered here. Further, Halliday's description accounts for the transition from preverbal to verbal development and does not attempt to describe child communication within the boundaries of adult meaning. Essentially, Halliday directly observed a child's emerging communication and formulated hypotheses conerning the social language functions. He described a total of seven language functions, which are, in order of emergence, as follows:

1. INSTRUMENTAL, in which language is used to satisfy material needs.
2. REGULATORY, in which language is used to control actions of other persons.
3. INTERACTIONAL, in which language is used to establish and maintain contact with other persons.
4. PERSONAL, in which language is used to inform others of one's own behavior.
5. HEURISTIC, in which language is used to explore and obtain explanations about the environment.
6. IMAGINATIVE, in which language is used to create a pretend environment.
7. INFORMATIVE, in which language is used to give information to someone who it is believed did not possess the information.

The first three functions, termed pragmatic, are interpersonal in nature, and generally relate to using communication to act upon the environment. These functions, as such, require some sort of response from the environment. The remaining functions, termed mathetic, are ideational in nature and represent the use of communication to code experiences. The informative function, which emerges significantly later than the others, is the one that indicates that the child is using language in the adult sense, or engaging in true language. The mastery of the other six functions is regarded as necessary for true language production.

Overall, Halliday has suggested that children learn, and with prespeech communicative forms, convey these meanings (excepting the informative) well before they have a conventional verbal means of expression. These social meanings then provide the foundation for the later expression of conventional language forms.

Initially, children learn the interpersonal nature of communication. After they have begun to express various interpersonal functions, they then differentiate the interpersonal from the ideational, and express functions in one mode (interpersonal or ideational) or the other. At this point there is no longer a one-to-one correspondence between a communication and a function. Rather, a communication may be used to express more than one function.

Halliday's description of prespeech and early verbal communication has important clinical applications. For the professional working with a nonverbal or low-verbal disordered child, it provides a means of assessing the current status of communication. Specifically, the clinician can ascertain whether a child understands the interpersonal nature of communication by noting nonverbal use of the instrumental, regulatory, and interactional functions. Such an assessment is particularly important for treatment programming. If a child does not understand that communication can be used to act upon the environment, then the establishment of such would be prerequisite to verbal intervention.

Environmental Communicative Input

As investigators have examined the role of input language, it has become clear that there are a number of ways in which input may influence, either positively or negatively, the language acquisition process (Cross, 1978; Gleason & Weintraub, 1978; Nelson, 1973). Although there are still many gray areas with respect to the influences of input, some general statements can be made.

It has been well documented that adults modify speech addressed to young children (Cross, 1977; Gleason & Weintraub, 1978; Lieven, 1978; Newhoff, Silverman & Millet, 1980; Newport, Gleitman, & Gleitman, 1977; Snow, 1972, 1977). However, the reason why such modifications might occur is not entirely clear. Some researchers have suggested that input is modified so as to teach children language. Others have suggested that teaching is not the primary goal, rather, the input is modified to achieve communication with children on their level. Still others have suggested that the input is modified so as to maintain a flow of conversation with children, therefore providing an appropriate model of conversational exchanges. Gleason and Weintraub (1978) have suggested that input plays different roles according to the age of the child. They described input to children under 12 months of age as serving primarily to establish an affectional bond. Input to children learning language (12 to 48 months) was viewed as facilitatory with respect to abstraction of linguistic knowledge. Finally, input to children over four years of age was characterized as providing information about the world.

There appears to be no clear agreement as to why children receive a specialized form of input. From the input literature, however, it is possible to extract those types of input that seem to exert a positive influence on the language-acquisition process. These are summarized in Table 4-1. As can be seen in the table, the first type of input described relates to expansions. It appears that expansions preserving a child's semantic intent exert a positive influence on language acquisition (Cross, 1977, 1978). Such expansions can occur in the form of noun phrase, pronoun, or verb phrase expansions. Examples of each of these forms of expansions can be seen in the table.

Table 4-1
Adult interactive strategies exerting positive influences on child language behavior.

1. **Comments in the form of expansions preserving a child's semantic intent.**
   a. Noun phrase expansions: An utterance incorporating the noun phrase topic.

   > Child: *kitty jump*
   > Adult: *the kitty is on the chair*

   b. Pronoun expansions: An utterance that incorporates the child's topic by using pronominalization.

   > Child: *kitty jump*
   > Adult: *she is jumping*

   c. Verb phrase expansions: An utterance preserving the topic expressed by the child in the verb phrase, but using a lexical item not found in the child's noun phrase.

   > Child: *kitty jump*
   > Adult: *the dog is jumping, too*

2. **Allowing the child to select the topic of joint (i.e., adult-child) attention.**

3. **Feedback responding to the truth value of a child's utterance, rather than linguistic accuracy.**

   > Child: *kitty jump*
   > Adult: *yes, the kitty is jumping*

A second factor in adult-child interaction that can influence language acquisition pertains to synchrony of the adult with the child's level. Specifically, children gain the most verbally when the adult is in cognitive as well as verbal synchrony with the child. Behaviorally, such synchrony can be facilitated by allowing the child to take the lead and, therefore, direct the activity or interaction.

This particular input variable becomes especially important when we consider the nature of most current treatment procedures. In many treatment programs, a child is presented with stimuli previously selected by the clinician. These stimuli may be objects or pictures that the clinician perceives as being within the child's conceptual abilities; but, in fact, there is the risk of a mismatch with respect to adult-child synchrony. The risk is particularly high in early language intervention, as it is apparent from the normal literature that an adult meaning system cannot be imposed on child language. It may be that in a situation in which the clinician has selected the stimuli, and the child is making minimal progress in treatment, the stimuli selected by the clinician are simply beyond the child's conceptual level. By allowing the child to select the topic of joint attention, it cannot be guaranteed that a mismatch in synchrony will not occur. Rather, the assumption is made that if the child is allowed to take the lead, it further reduces the possiblility of a mismatch that may impede treatment progress.

Nelson (1977) has examined the influences of these first two input variables in the language of normal children. In this study, an experimenter engaged in play with the children. During the play sessions, semantically related expansions of the children's preceding utterances were provided. The utterance types modeled by the experimenter (in the form of expansions) represented syntactic structures not used by the children at the initiation of the study. Following termination of experimental procedures, the children were observed to use the modeled syntactic forms. It was concluded that the procedures resulted in the acquisition of new syntactic forms by the children.

The final input variable to be discussed relates to the way adults respond to children's utterances. Children seem to derive maximum benefit from input that responds to the truth value, rather than the linguistic accuracy, of their utterances. This point has been discussed by various investigators (Bowerman, 1976; Bruner, 1975; Nelson, 1973). Nelson noted that there are some mothers who function in a directive mode and seemingly attempt to teach their children correct words. In doing such, they were observed to correct their children's inacccurate productions. Nelson concluded that this style of interaction slowed the children's language learning. Bruner, in his studies of mother-child interaction, supported Nelson's view of negative feedback. He suggested that maternal corrections have an undesirable effect on the communicative interaction. Bowerman provided a detailed discussion on the role of negative feedback in language acquisition. Following a review of various studies, she suggested that "feedback about inadequate performance is neither required for language learning nor does it particularly accelerate its pace" (1976, p. 170).

This rather ominous view of negative feedback has important implications for treatment procedures currently practiced with language-disordered children. Clearly, many treatment procedures rely on correction of inaccurate responses. In view of current information relative to negative feedback, this mode of treatment should probably be modified. However, as Bowerman has pointed out, most information relative to the role of negative feedback has been derived from normal populations. It may be that with disordered children, who have obviously not acquired language in a normal manner, negative, as well as positive, feedback is necessary for the accurate formulation of linguistic hypotheses.

Conversational Conventions

Another aspect of communicative competence relates to the ability to engage appropriately in a communicative interaction. Such appropriateness goes beyond the individual utterance level and focuses more on conversatioinal behaviors. Generally, three basic skills are required in order to engage in a socially appropriate conversational interaction. As described by Wilcox and Webster (1980), they are (1) the initiation and maintenance of a communicative interaction, (2) consideration of the listener's perspective when encoding messages, and (3) appropriate responses to listener feedback. Initiation and maintenance of an interaction relies heavily on nonverbal behavior, such as gaze regulation, use of silences, timing of speech, and turn-taking. Consideration of the listener's perspective requires awareness of shared, as well as unshared, information between speaker and listener. Appropriate responses to listener feedback require answering questions and appropriately repeating or recoding utterances as indicated by the listener feedback.

Numerous investigators have examined the development of communicative conventions in normal children (Gallagher, 1977; Garvey, 1977; Wellman & Lempers, 1977; Wilcox & Webster, 1980). In general, evidence indicates that children have a basic understanding of these skills by age four. Further, it has been suggested that these skills may function independently of the level of linguistic development. Clinically, this means that an evaluation of linguistic skills is not sufficient to ascertain functioning in terms of communicative competence. Assessment procedures should also include provisions to evaluate children's awareness of socially appropriate communicative conventions.

The need for evaluating both aspects (i.e., linguistic as well as socially appropriate interpersonal skills) of a child's communication is further substantiated in a recent study by Blank, Gessner, and Esposito (1979). The investigation consisted of the analysis of the communicative behavior of a child (age 3;3) while interacting with his parents over a 10-week period. The child was initially referred for an evaluation because of his refusal to interact with anyone other than his parents. Analysis of the linguistic aspects of the child's speech (e.g., semantic relations and syntax) revealed age-appropriate behavior. However, analysis of the child's interpersonal communicative functioning revealed numerous difficulties. Most noticable was his inability to use or comprehend gestures (e.g., pointing) or to appropriately respond to utterances. His responses, when made, were usually irrelevant to the preceding comment.

Communicative Competence: Studies with Language-Disordered Children

Communicative Functions

One of the first investigations of language-disordered children's use of communicative functions was conducted by Snyder (1975). Her participants included 15 language-disordered and 15 normal children, all functioning at the one-word stage of language production. The children were presented with tasks designed to elicit imperative and declarative functions. Responses were scored on a five-point scale ranging from nonverbal to verbal behavior. On both function measures, the language-disordered children produced fewer verbal functions, and were observed to engage in more nontask responses than the normal children.

In a more recent investigation, Leonard, Camarata, Rowan, and Chapman (1982) also examined the communicative functions of young language-disordered children. The participants in the study included 14 normal and 14 language-impaired children. Both groups of children were functioning at the single-word stage of language production. Spontaneous language samples were obtained from all children and were then analyzed using McShane's (1980) classification of communicative functions. The classification system included the following major functions:

1. **Regulation**—attempts to control other persons' behaviors
2. **Statement**—utterances that name, describe, or provide information about a situation not in the here and now
3. **Exchange**—utterances made when a child is giving or receiving objects from another person
4. **Personal**—utterances about what the child is doing, or about to be doing, as well as refusals and protests
5. **Conversation**—utterances in response to preceding utterances produced by other people.

Results indicated that the groups of children were highly similar in their use of the functions with two exceptions. The normal children produced more statement functions in the form of naming, while the language-disordered children produced more conversation functions in the form of answering. Since statement functions are child-initiated, while the conversation functions are not, it could be said that the language-disordered children were less likely to spontaneously initiate verbal communications.

In another recent investigation, communicative functions served by echolalic behavior in autistic children was examined (Prizant & Duchan, 1981). Four children diagnosed as autistic, and ranging in age from 4;8 to 9;3, were videotaped in a variety of natural settings. Of particular interest were the children's echolalic utterances. By viewing such utterances in their natural contexts, the authors posited seven different functions the echoic utterances seemed to be serving. The majority of the children's echoic utterances fell into four categories that appeared to be communicative in nature. These included turn-taking, declaration, affirmation, and request.

These preceding studies of communicative functions produced by language-disordered children contain a wealth of information applicable to the treatment process. First, they provide guidelines for assessment and treatment by specifically identifying various communicative functions. Second, they alert one to the possibility that there may be differences in language-disordered children's use of functions as compared to normals. Finally, the study by Prizant and Duchan importantly emphasizes the need to evaluate the communicative use of behaviors that are frequently regarded by clinicians as undesirable and noncommunicative in nature.

Conversational Skills

Another important aspect of language-disordered children's communicative competence pertains to their conversational functioning beyond the level of expressing functions. These aspects of communication are frequently referred to as discourse abilities and include behaviors mentioned in the first section of this chapter. These are (1) initiating and sustaining a communicative interaction, (2) considering a listener's perspective when encoding messages, and (3) responding to listener feedback.

Initiation of a communicative interaction involves obtaining attention and then asserting the desired message. Typically, initiation comprises nonverbal behaviors, such as eye contact and body position, as its first steps. For example, to initiate an interaction, a potential speaker will usually look at, then lean or walk toward, a potential listener. If necessary, these nonverbal behaviors may be supplemented, especially in young children, by verbal attention-getters, such as "Hey, " "Look, " or by producing the name of the person whose attention is desired.

Investigators who have examined initiation abilities of language-disordered children have suggested that appropriate initiation skills may represent a problem area (Dukes, 1981; Lucas, 1980). It appears that some language-disordered children not only have difficulty appropriately obtaining attention for purposes of initiation, but they also attempt to initiate communication at inappropriate times. Further, it has been suggested that once attention has been obtained, some children with language disorders may have difficulty asserting their desired message for reasons unrelated to their linguistic deficits. Hence, potential problems with initiation may be at the verbal (asserting a message) or nonverbal (eye contact, body posture) level.

The ability to sustain a communicative interaction involves a variety of behaviors. These include turn-taking conventions, the production of utterances appropriate and relevant to preceding utterances, acknowledgement and/or answers to questions, and requests for clarification of ambiguous messages. Various studies have found deficits in language-disordered children with respect to these abilities (Donahue, Pearl, & Bryan, 1980; Dukes, 1981; Lucas, 1980; Miller, 1978). Language-disordered children have been observed to violate turn-taking conventions, produce irrelevant utterances, ignore questions, and, infrequently, request clarification of ambiguous or nonunderstood messages. In general it can be said that some language-disordered children may have problems maintaining control of a communicative interaction for a sufficient length of time to express a desired message.

Another aspect of conversational proficiency relates to the consideration of a listener's perspective when encoding utterances. Basically, this means that a speaker must be able to integrate verbal and contextual information in such a way that the utterance produced is as informative as the situation requires. The degree of speaker informativeness required will depend on different factors. One factor pertains to a speaker's awareness of information already available to, or shared by, a listener. Such information can be apparent from linguistic or nonlinguistic context. A second factor pertains to a speaker's awareness of listener limitations that may require modifications of his or her normal communicative behavior.

Although little research has focused on young language-disordered children's abilities to consider a listener's perspective, there are two recent studies relating to aspects of this skill. Shatz, Bernstein, and Shulman (1980) examined language-disordered children's responses to indirect directives (e.g., "Can you put the dolly in the bed?"). Utterances such as these are frequently referred to as indirect requests. For example, "Can you put the dolly in the bed?" is literally a question about one's ability to perform the stated action. If a listener had both arms in casts, then a literal interpretation of this utterance would be appropriate. However, in a context in which there are no apparent limitations on a listener's mobility—which is to say that listener's mobility is shared information—then the utterance would be regarded as a request to perform the stated action. Thus, appropriate interpretations of utterances coded in an indirect format rely on the listener's ability to compare the utterance with the context in which it is produced.

Shatz et al. examined aspects of language-disordered children's abilities to encode context by noting their responses to indirect, as well as direct, sentence forms. In the study, five language-disordered children ranging in age from 5 to 6 years served as participants. In an initial experiment, the children were seen in a familiar therapy room equipped with toys, and presented with direct ("Put the ball in the truck. ") and indirect ("Can you put the ball in the truck?") requests. Results indicated that the children performed the requested action the majority of the time.

A second experiment was conducted that more specifically examined the children's abilities to consider contextual cues. In this experiment, the children were presented with test utterances only in the *can* + *you* format. However, this time the utterances were preceded by verbal information designed to foster either (1) literal interpretation of the utterance as a question ("Can you run fast?") or (2) interpretation of the utterance as a request ("Can you give me the toy?"). Results indicated the the children had difficulty using the information given in the prior linguistic context, particularly when the context indicated that the appropriate interpretation would be as a question.

Fey, Leonard, and Wilcox (1981) examined language-disordered children's abilities to modify their speech as a function of listener age. Six language-disordered children, ranging in age from 4;3 to 6;5 served as participants. The participants were observed in a free-play setting with (1) a language-normal child of the same age and (2) a language-normal child who was younger, but exhibited linguistic abilities similar to the disordered child. The results indicated that the participants simplified their speech somewhat when communicating with the younger children. Specifically, they exhibited a shorter mean preverb length, while also using more sentence forms designed to engage the younger children in an interaction.

At this time, general conclusions cannot be drawn with respect to language-disordered children's abilities to consider a listener's perspective. It would be most prudent to say that perspective-taking, as described previously, is an important skill for effective communication. It may constitute a problem area for some children, especially when they are required to evaluate prior linguistic context.

The final aspect of conversational proficiency to be discussed concerns responses to listener feedback indicating a lack of understanding. More specifically, a speaker must be able to provide clarification of utterances that a listener has indicated are ambiguous. Some research has focused on this ability in language-disordered children. Gallagher and Darnton (1978) examined these children's attempts to clarify their utterances in response to the question "What?" Results indicated that the majority of the time, the children recoded their original utterances.

Pearl, Donahue, and Bryan (1979) also examined language-disordered children's responses to clarification requests. The children were provided with three types of feedback, (1) explicit ("Tell me more") (2) implicit ("I don't understand"), and (3) facial feedback which consisted of a puzzled look. Results indicated that the children attempted to clarify utterances in response to all types of feedback.

From research conducted thus far, it would appear that language-disordered children recognize the need to clarify ambiguous messages. However, the degree to which their clarifications are successful has yet to be determined. Hence, the ability to clarify an ambiguous utterance successfully also merits consideration for potential treatment content.

The Integration of Communicative Competence into Early Language Intervention: An Exemplary Treatment Model

As a professional concerned with the management of language-disordered children, my primary interest in studies of the nature of children's communication is their application to the treatment process for disordered populations. Throughout the first two sections of this chapter, as well as in the chapter by Leonard (this volume), brief suggestions were made in this regard. As is all too often the case with disordered populations, specific studies of the treatment process are relatively few in number. Further, as the idea of communicative competence is relatively new, the number of available references is even further reduced (Leonard, 1981). Hence, a specialist who recognizes the need to improve a child's communicative, rather than purely linguistic, competence must frequently review the literature and then develop his or her own procedures.

It is my intent to devote the remainder of this chapter to a discussion of the ways in which the literature I have previously reviewed can be applied to the treatment process. To accomplish this, I will present, in detail, an exemplary treatment model for preschool language intervention. The model is not intended to be all-inclusive. Rather, it illustrates one way in which aspects of linguistic, as well as communicative, competence can be treated.

In the more recent literature, there are other treatment procedures reflecting current trends in the study of child language. Taenzer, Cermak, and Hanlon (1981), as well as Culotta and Horn (1982), describe procedures that incorporate important pragmatic variables or modify spontaneous communicative behavior. Dukes (1981) outlines an approach based on group activities that focuses on several aspects of communicative competence, including nonverbal as well as verbal skills. Finally, Lucas (1980) describes procedures oriented toward the appropriate use of linguistic forms in social settings.

The treatment model to be discussed here incorporates several of the parameters of communicative competence addressed in previous sections of this chapter. First, the importance of prespeech communication is recognized by including procedures designed to establish social language functions expressed during prespeech communication. Second, input behaviors found to have a positive influence on language acquisition are utilized in the intervention procedures. Specifically, these include (a) semantically related expansions of child utterances, (b) child-directed interactions, and (c) clinician feedback responding to the truth value of child utterances. Third, to enable modification of spontaneous communicative behavior, treatment takes place in a free-play setting in which few restrictions are placed on the child's verbal or nonverbal behavior. By staging the treatment setting in this manner, children's utterances are not treated in isolation. Rather, the focus of treatment is on conversational competence. This setting also allows the clinician to model socially appropriate communicative conventions (i.e., initiating and sustaining a communicative interaction, consideration of a listener's perspective, and appropriate responses to listener feedback).

The treatment protocol is divided into three phases. The first phase is referred to as nonverbal intervention. This phase is designed to establish intentional communication in the form of gestures and/or vocalizations. The second phase establishes initial verbal skills in the form of a core lexicon. The final phase focuses on expansion of verbal skills beyond the single-word level. Each of these phases will be considered separately.

Nonverbal Intervention

This first part of the protocol is designed for children who do not understand the interpersonal nature of communication. Typically, such children exhibit no identifiable forms of intentional communication. The assumption is made that the ability to manipulate the environment intentionally is necessary for language development. Hence, the goal at this phase of intervention, which is based upon Halliday's (1975) model of language acquisition, is to establish the following social meanings: interactional, instrumental, and regulatory. These meanings will then serve as the basis for later conventional expressions.

The procedures and goals for this initial intervention are summarized in Table 4-2. Upon completion of this phase of the protocol, a child will (1) understand that communication can be used to obtain attention and (2) understand that communication can be used to obtain assistance in achieving desired ends. Operationally, this translates into the goals listed in Table 4-2. Although the interactional function appears first in the outline, it is not necessarily trained first. In reality all three functions (interactional, instrumental, and regulatory) can be the focus of training at the same time.

The first step in establishing the interactional function requires the clinician to attend to the child's behavior and comment about the child's activity or focus of attention. At this point, the basic idea is for the child to begin to understand that his or her activities are of interest to the clinician. Over time, this adult interest will take on the properties of a reinforcer for the child. The child will in turn start engaging in behaviors to obtain attention from the clinician.

At this step of intervention, it is critical that the clinician follow the child's lead. This means that no attempts should be made to direct the play activities, other than imposing limits on potentially harmful behaviors. The clinician, by behaving in this essentially nondirective fashion, is facilitating adult-child synchrony. In this way, the clinician's comments, which can be regarded as verbal expansions of the child's nonverbal interactions, are more likely to be within the child's conceptual sphere. Clinician comments about the child's activities should be of a simple linguistic form, generally at the single- or two-word utterance level.

Eventually, the clinician will begin to place contingencies on the child that concern his or her attending behavior. However, at least three unconditional sessions are initially required. The actual number of such sessions will vary depending on how frequently the child is seen for treatment. For example, if a child is seen for treatment on an infrequent basis (i.e., once a week) a larger number of unconditional sessions will probably be required.

After the initial unconditional sessions, the clinician can begin placing contingencies on attending. Attention is therefore withheld in an attempt to elicit some form of appropriate attention-getting behavior from the child. The actual behaviors to be evoked will vary from child to child, and should be predetermined by the clinician. Generally, appropriate attention-getting behavior will take the form of eye contact or gestures which may or may not be accompanied by a vocalization.

As the clinician begins to place contingencies on attending, the child may initially make no attempt to get attention from the clinician. If this

Table 4-2
Nonverbal intervention.

1. **Interactional Function**
   Goal: Establish appropriate attention-getting behavior
   a. Attend to child's behavior and comment
   b. Place contingencies on giving attention
2. **Instrumental/Regulatory Function**
   Goal: Establish a clear signal indicating assistance is required
   a. Anticipate need for assistance, and comply
   b. Place contingencies on providing assistance

occurs, the clinician should return to the first step for a session and continue to probe by periodically witholding attention. As the child initially begins to make attempts to obtain attention, she or he may exhibit very slight moving-toward behaviors. Such behaviors should be noted, reinforced with attention, and then incorporated into a procedure of successive approximation to achieve the desired end goal.

The establishment of the instrumental and regulatory functions also relies on the clinician following the child's lead and then verbally expanding the child's nonverbal interactions. In the case of these functions, the procedures initially require the clinician to anticipate a child's need for assistance, and comply. For example, the child may be looking at a toy on a high shelf. The clinician would then get the toy and give it to the child, while making a comment such as "here."

As with the interactional function, at least three sessions should be unconditional. It is initially necessary to establish the pattern that the clinician can, and is willing to, assist the child. After the initial unconditional sessions, the clinician can begin to place contingencies on providing his or her assistance. Specifically, the clinician does not provide assistance until the child makes some attempt to engage it. Again, the process of successive approximation should be employed to establish the desired target response.

Once these interpersonal functions have been established a child is ready to begin initial verbal intervention. To determine such readiness, a productivity criterion is used. That is, a child is required to demonstrate productive use of the interpersonal communicative functions (interactional and instrumental and/or regulatory). A function is regarded as being productive if it is expressed in at least five different contexts during a given treatment session. To ensure a degree of stability, two consecutive probes meeting this criterion are required.

Productivity, rather than percentage of use was selected as a criterion as percentages can often be misleading. A child may be producing a function 90% of the time. However, if that function is always in the same context it may be that a child has not actually acquired the communicative behavior in a manner that is useful for communication. That is to say that the child may not have acquired a generalizable communicative behavior. Thus, in keeping treatment data, percentages are still recorded but productive use of a behavior is used for purposes of determining acquisition.

Table 4-3 displays data on a child who was exposed to this initial phase of intervention. The female child was 3;10 at the time of intervention. The initial diagnostic evaluation revealed no verbal communication and little-to-no nonverbal communication. Parental reports confirmed the diagnostic impressions. Initial baseline observations were conducted to assess percentage of time spent engaging in the interpersonal communicative functions as well as the number of different contexts in which the functions were expressed. Interpersonal communications were identified as those instances in which the child sought the attention or assistance of the clinician. Three baseline observations were made via videotape. During this time the clinician and the child were in a large room equipped with various age-appropriate toys. The clinician was instructed to "engage in play with the child." Each baseline session was thirty minutes in duration.

The videotapes were reviewed and the duration of each interpersonal communicative act was timed. The percentage of time spent engaging in interpersonal communication as well as the number of different contexts was then computed for the child. Once the baseline data were obtained, treatment began. The child was seen four times weekly in individual treatment that was thirty minutes in duration.

The child was initially exposed to three unconditional treatment sessions. Contingencies were then placed on the clinician's attention and compliance during the fourth session. The data displayed in Table 4-3, therefore, represent the baseline information, the first three unconditional treatment sessions, and weekly probes. As can be seen from the Table, the child reached criterion during the fourth week of treatment. Treatment was extended for an additional week to ensure stability.

Initial Verbal Intervention

This phase of the treatment protocol is designed for children who exhibit intentional communication, but do not code it in conventional terms. The general idea is to establish a core lexicon. Various investigators (e.g.,

Table 4-3
Data: Nonverbal intervention.

Session Type	% Time Engaged Interpersonal Communication Functions	Number of Different Contexts	
		Interactional	Regulatory/ Instrumental
Baseline	08	1	1
Baseline	06	1	1
Baseline	09	1	1
Treatment No. 1 (no contingencies)	12	1	2
Treatment No. 2 (no contingencies)	10	1	2
Treatment No. 3 (no contingencies)	11	1	2
Weekly Probe No. 1 (contingencies)	20	2	3
Weekly Probe No. 2 (contingencies)	24	2	2
Weekly Probe No. 3 (contingencies)	39	4	3
Weekly Probe No. 4 (contingencies)	51	5	5
Weekly Probe No. 5 (contingencies)	56	6	5

Bowerman, 1976; Holland, 1975) have provided guidelines for selection of such a core, and the reader is referred to them for purposes of devising an appropriate initial lexicon. The primary focus of this section will be on procedures for establishing whatever core lexicon has been selected. The procedures for this phase of intervention are summarized in Table 4-4.

The initial lexicon is trained in the context of the interactional, instrumental, and regulatory functions. As with the first phase of the protocol, there is no order to the establishment of the functions. Rather, the context dictates what particular function will be verbally coded.

The general procedures for establishing the initial words are very similar to the procedures outlined for establishing the interpersonal functions in phase 1 of the protocol. The actual steps to be followed are listed in Table 4-4. As can be seen, the clinician's attention and assistance are serving as the means for establishing the target words. A child either beginning, or moving into, this second phase of the protocol already understands the interpersonal communicative functions, and, as such, can be regarded as motivated to communicate. Essentially, in this second phase of treatment, the child will begin mapping conventional verbal signs upon interpersonal functions that are already in use.

As with phase 1 of the protocol, the initial treatment sessions should be conducted with no contingencies. Thus, for at least three sessions, the clinician will follow the child's lead and expand the nonverbal communicative acts in the form of words from the core lexicon. Hence, all clinician comments will initially be in the form of a single-word utterance. Following these unconditional sessions, the clinician may then begin to introduce contingencies in the forms of steps 2 and 3 (appearing in Table 4-4). The intermediate step, in which any vocalization is accepted, is necessary only for those children who do not accompany their nonverbal communications with vocalizations. Since many children will spontaneously do this while expressing social functions (Halliday, 1975), this step will not be necessary for all children.

In terms of size of the core lexicon, it is recommended that 10 to 15 words be initially selected. As with phase 1 of the protocol a productivity criteria is employed. Specifically, when a child is using a given lexical item in at least five different contexts, he or she is regarded as ready to incorporate that item in more complex linguistic structures.

Table 4-5 displays data obtained from a child who was exposed to this second phase of the treatment protocol. The data is in percentage form so as to display an overall picture of the types of communicative behaviors. The male child was aged 2;10 at the initiation of treatment. The diagnostic evaluation revealed intentional communication expressed primarily with gestural symbols. The only conventional linguistic sign was 'mama." This

Table 4-4
Initial Verbal Intervention

1. **Interactional Function**
   a. Child demonstrates attention-getting behavior, clinician attends and provides word for joint focus of attention.
   b. Contingencies placed on attending: Clinician withholds attention until child pairs nonverbal signal with a vocalization. Clinician then attends and provides word for joint focus of attention.
   c. Contingencies placed on attending: Clinician withholds attention until child utilizes word (or acceptable approximation). Clinician then attends and expands with two-word utterance.

2. **Instrumental/Regulatory Function**
   a. Child produces signal for assistance, clinician provides assistance and produces word.
   b. Contingencies placed on providing assistance: Clinician doesn't assist until child pairs nonverbal signal with a vocalization. Clinician then complies and produces desired word.
   c. Contingencies placed on providing assistance: Clinician doesn't assist until child uses word (or acceptable approximation). Clinician then complies and expands with a two-word utterance.

sign was regarded as productive. Parental reports confirmed the findings in the diagnostic evaluation.

The child was seen for individual treatment four times weekly. Each session was thirty minutes long. Baseline information was obtained for the first three sessions via videotape. During baseline collection, the clinician was simply instructed to "engage in play with the child." The tapes were reviewed and the communicative acts were coded with respect to (1) the social language function and (2) the means used to express the function. The interactional, instrumental, and regulatory functions were consistently used. The means of expression were coded as gestural, gesture and vocalization, single-word utterances, and two-word utterances. Percentages in each of these categories were computed. The baseline information appearing in the table represents the mean of these sessions. Additionally, contexts of each word production were noted (e.g., "truck" while pushing the truck; "truck" while pointing to a truck out of reach). These notations then served as the basis for determining word productivity.

Following baseline, treatment procedures began. The goal was to establish a core lexicon of at least 15 words. Weekly probes were obtained by video recording during the last treatment session in each week. During the fourth week, the established criterion was met for seven of the target words. At this point, the clinician began modeling two word utterances incorporating these words while she continued to model single word responses for those words that were not yet productive. The effects of this can be seen with the resulting increases in two-word responses. These expanded child responses incorporated the productive lexical items.

Expansion of Verbal Skills

This phase of the protocol is designed for children who are ready to expand verbal skills beyond the single-word level. The procedures in this phase can be used to establish use of semantic relations, grammatical morphemes, kernel-sentence structures, or transformational structures. The specific target selected simply varies according to a child's needs. To determine the appropriate target structure, it is recommended that a spontaneous language sample be obtained and analyzed. Miller (1981) has several suggestions and recommendations for the specifics of such an analysis. Once the analyses of the language sample have been done, it is recommended that the clinician consult developmental norms for purposes of determining appropriate target responses for the child.

In terms of specific procedures, as with phases 1 and 2 of the protocol, it is important for the clinician to follow the child's lead. To facilitate this, the clinician should engage in imitative play. This means that the clinician watches the child and then plays in exactly the same way as she or he does. For example, if a child begins stacking blocks, the clinician will also stack blocks. With many children, this imitative play will not be necessary, as the children themselves will specify what they want the clinician to do. For example, a child may be engaging in a pretend cooking activity in which he will give the clinician instructions such as, "Put the plate there" or "Pour the milk now," and so on. So the general rule is for the clinician to engage in imitative play unless otherwise specified by the child.

The other two input facilitators appearing in Table 4-1 of this chapter are also used by the clinician. Specifically, the clinician expands child utterances in the form of the selected target response and, when a child uses the target response, responds to the truth value. Table 4-6 summarizes the steps and procedures for this phase of the protocol. As can be seen upon examining the table, when the child makes a comment, the clinician expands with the target response. If the child is quiet, the clinician will code the

Table 4-5
Data: Initial verbal intervention.

Session	Gesture %	Gesture and Vocalization %	Single-Word %	Two-Word %
Baseline	91	05	04	00
Week 1[1]	90	03	07	00
Week 2[2]	51	19	30	00
Week 3	52	15	33	00
Week 4	25	18	56	00
Week 5[3]	16	14	70	00
Week 6	11	19	65	05
Week 7	07	10	65	18

[1]No contingencies placed on clinician attention and assistance
[2]Contingencies placed on clinician attention and assistance
[3]Clinician began modeling two-word utterances for productive lexical items

nonverbal behavior in the form of the target response. If the child produces the target response, the clincian will confirm the truth value and expand one level beyond the target response. Essentially, unless the child actually produces the target response, all clinician verbal behavior will be in the form of the desired target response.

The criterion for acquisition of a given structure varies as a function of the selected target response. If a target behavior is a grammatical morpheme, the criterion for termination of treatment is 50% usage in obligatory contexts for two consecutive treatment sessions. A relatively liberal criterion is employed because experience with the protocol has indicated that at a time in which children are using a grammatical morpheme during 50% of the required contexts, they have, in effect, acquired the structure and are able to stablize use on their own. However, once criterion has been reached, the clinician should monitor the structure for a few sessions. If there appears to be a pattern of decreased use, then that structure should again be the focus of treatment.

If the target behavior is a semantic relation, kernel structure, or transformation, the same criterion used in phases 1 and 2 is employed. However,

Table 4-6
Expansion of verbal skills.

1. **Identify verbal target (e.g., agent + action)**
2. **Child initiates activity and clinician imitates play unless otherwise specified by the child.**
3. **Clinician verbal behavior:**
   a. If child makes a comment, the clinician expands in the form of the verbal target.

   Child: *doggie* (as making dog jump)
   Clinician: *doggie jump* (while also making dog jump)

   b. If child is quiet, the clinician does the nonverbal behavior in the form of the target structure.

   Child: making dog jump
   Clinician: doggie jump (while also making dog jump)

   c. If child produces target structure, the clinician responds to the truth value, then expands the utterance.

   Child: *doggie jump*
   Clinician: *yes, doggie jumping*

productivity is defined in terms of word combinations rather than non-linguistic contexts. Specifically, a given structure is regarded as productive if it occurs at least five times in combination with different words for two consecutive treatment sessions.

Since all treatment sessions take place in a free play, spontaneous context, it is not necessary to gather additional samples for purposes of determining whether criterion has been reached. The clinician is, in fact, treating spontaneous speech. Hence, an analysis of the child's language used during a treatment session will yield the desired information. To chart a given child's progress, it is recommended that weekly analyses be conducted.

Table 4-7 displays data from a child exposed to this phase of the treatment protocol. The male child was age 3;8 at the initiation of treatment. His mean length of response in morphemes was 2.29. The initial treatment goal was to establish productive use of the subject + verb + object (SVO) sentence structure. Once productivity of this structure was acquired, the goal was to establish use of the present progressive within the same kernel structure. Hence, data on both structures was recorded from the outset of treatment. Although the table displays percentage of use, productivity as previously defined was the criterion employed.

Table 4-7
Results of expansion of subject + verb + object (SVO) skills.

Session	SVO %	SVing0 %
Baseline	01	00
Week 1	02	00
Week 3	20	00
Week4[1]	24	00
Week 5	28	14
Week 6	30	20
Week 7[2]	35	34

[1]SVO was productive during this weekly probe

[2]SVing0 was productive during this weekly probe

The child was seen twice weekly for treatment. Each treatment session was one and one-half hours in duration and consisted of individual and group treatment. For the first four weeks of treatment the clinician modeled only the SVO sentence structure. Analysis of the sample obtained during the fourth week indicated that the structure was productive. The clinician then began modeling the SVO sentence structure with the present progressive form. This structure was productive during the seventh week of treatment.

Orazi (1981) also conducted a study analyzing the effectiveness of phase three of the treatment protocol. The subjects consisted of seven language-disordered children. The children ranged in age from 3;5 to 4;7 at the initiation of treatment. They ranged in mean length of utterance in morphemes from 2.52 to 4.70. All children demonstrated absence of use of the yes/no question transformation upon analyses of spontaneous language samples. For purposes of evaluating treatment effectiveness, children were assigned to either an experimental or control group. Thus, four children received treatment and three received no treatment. Those assigned to the experimental group were exposed to treatment, designed to establish use of the yes/no question transformation, until productivity of the structure was obtained. Once they met criterion, experimental-control comparisons were made. The experimental group demonstrated significant gains in the target structure as compared to the control group.

Summary and Conclusions

Several recent trends in the child language literature that have important implications for preschool language disorders have been considered. These include the relationship of prespeech communication to later verbal communication, the role of environmental communicative input in children's language acquisition, and young children's knowledge with respect to socially appropriate communicative conventions.

A developmentally based treatment protocol has been discussed. The protocol is designed for preschool language-disordered children. The procedures incorporate adult behaviors found to have a positive influence on child language behavior. The protocol further includes provisions to establish, if necessary, socio-communicative knowledge regarded as necessary for verbal development. The remaining phases of the protocol include procedures for establishing an initial lexicon and, then, expansion of the lexicon in terms of semantic relations, kernel sentences, grammatical morphemes, and transformations.

Through presentation of data at each phase of the protocol, it can be seen that the procedures are effective in establishing the desired behaviors. However, there are aspects of the procedures that require further evaluation. First, the clinician is, in effect, treating spontaneous speech. Therefore, the assumption is made that generalization is, in fact, occurring outside the treatment setting. However, this assumption has not yet been verified. Second, it would be useful to determine whether the protocol can be utilized to establish social language functions other than the interactional, instrumental, and regulatory. It also seems possible that the protocol could serve as a basis for parent training. In instances where a clinician has a particularly large potential case load, explorations with adaptations of the model for parents might be a viable alternative to lengthy waiting lists. Finally, I want to again emphasize that this model serves only as one example of a treatment procedure focusing on the development of linguistic and communicative competence. In many cases, the clinician may be faced with a case in which she or he will rely on a mixture of approaches in order to achieve treatment goals.

Acknowledgments

I wish to thank Ann Grant-Harbin and Kay Halfhill for their assistance in gathering data on the treatment protocol. A special thanks is extended to Marilyn Newhoff for her input in development of the treatment protocol.

References

Barten, S. Development of gesture. In N. Smith & M. Franklin (Eds.), *Symbolic functioning in childhood.* Hillsdale, NJ: Lawrence Erlbaum, 1979.

Bates, E. *Language and context: The acquisition of pragmatics.* New York: Academic Press, 1976.

Bates, E., Camaioni, L., & Volterra, V. The acquisition of performatives prior to speech. In E. Ochs & B. Achieffelin (Eds.), *Developmental pragmatics.* New York: Academic Press, 1979.

Blank, M., Gessner, M., & Esposito, A. Language without communication: A case study. *Journal of Child Language,* 1979, *6,* 329-352.

Bowerman, M. Semantic factors in the acquisition of rules for word use and sentence construction. In D. Morehead & A. Morehead (Eds.), *Normal and deficient child language.* Baltimore: University Park Press, 1976.

Braine, M. The ontogeny of English phrase structures: The first phase. *Language,* 1963, *30,* 1-14.

Brown, R., Cazden, C., & Bellugi, U. The child's grammar from I to III. In C. Ferguson & D. Slobin (Eds.), *Studies in child language development.* New York: Holt, Rinehart & Winston, 1973.

Brown, R., & Hanlon, C. Derivational complexity and order of acquisition in child speech. In J. Hayes (Ed.) *Cognition and the development of language.* New York: Wiley, 1970.

Bruner, J. The ontogenesis of speech acts. *Journal of Child Language,* 1975, *2,* 1-19.

Bruner, J. Learning how to do things with words. In D. Aaronson & R. Reiber (Eds.), *Psycholinguistic research: Implications and applications.* Hillsdale, NJ: Lawrence Erlbaum, 1979.

Carter, A. From sensori-motor vocalizations to words: A case study in the evolution of attention-directing communication in the second year. In A. Lock (Ed.), *Action, gesture, and symbol.* New York: Academic Press, 1978.

Chomsky, N. *Syntactic structures.* Cambridge, MA: MIT Press, 1957.

Chomsky, N. *Aspects of a theory of syntax.* Cambridge, MA: MIT Press, 1965.

Clark, R. The transition from action to gesture. In A. Lock (Ed.), *Action, gesture, and symbol.* New York: Academic Press, 1978.

Cross, R. Mothers' speech adjustments: The control of selected child listener variables. In C. Snow & C. Ferguson (Eds.), *Talking to children: Language input and acquisition.* Cambridge, Eng: Cambridge University Press, 1977.

Cross, T. Mothers' speech and its association with rate of linguistic development in young children. In N. Waterson & C Snow (Eds.), *The development of communication.* New York: Wiley, 1978.

Culatta, B., & Horn, D. A program for generalization of grammatical rules to spontaneous discourse. *Journal of Speech and Hearing Disorders,* 1982, *47,* 174-180.

Dore, J. A pragmatic description of early development. *Journal of Psycholinguistic Research,* 1974, *3,* 343-350.

Donahue, M., Pearl, R., & Bryan, R. Conversational competence in learning disabled children: Responses to uninformative messsages, *Applied Psycholinguistics,* 1980, *1,* 387-403.

Dukes, P. Developing social prerequisites to oral communication. *Topics in Learning and Learning Disabilities,* 1981, *1,* 47-58.

Fey, M., Leonard, L., & Wilcox, K. Speech style modifications of language-impaired children. *Journal of Speech and Hearing Disorders,* 1981, *46,* 91-96.

Gallagher, T. Revision Behaviors in the speech of normal children developing language. *Journal of Speech and Hearing Research,* 1977, *20,* 303-318.

Gallagher, T., & Darnton, B. Conversational aspects of the speech of language-disordered children: Revision behaviors. *Journal of Speech and Hearing Research,* 1978, *21,*118-135.

Garvey, C. The contingent query: A dependent act in conversation. In M. Lewis & L. Rosenblum (Eds.), *Origins of behavior, Vol. 5: Communication and the development of language.* New York: Wiley, 1977.

Gleason, J. & Weintraub, S. Input language and the acquisition of communicative competence. In K. Nelson (Ed.), *Children's language: Vol. I.,* New York: Gardner Press, 1978.

Halliday, M. *Learning how to mean: Explorations in the development of language.* New York: Elsevier, 1975.

Holland, A. Language therapy for children: Some thoughts on context and content. *Journal of Speech and Hearing Disorders,* 1975, *40,* 514-523.

Hymes, D. Competence and performance in linguistic theory. In R. Huxley & E. Ingram (Eds.), *Language acquisition: Models and methods.* New York: Academic Press, 1971.

Lakoff, R. Language in context. *Language,* 1972, *48,* 907-927.

Leonard, L., Facilitating linguistic skills in children with specific language impairment. *Applied Psycholinguistics,* 1981, *2,* 89-118.

Leonard, L., Camarata, S., Rowan, L., & Chapman, D. The communicative functions of lexical usage by language-impaired children, *Applied Psycholinguistics,* 1982, *3,* 109-126

Lieven, E. Conversations between mothers and young children: Individual differences and their possible implication for the study of language learning. In N. Waterson & C. Snow (Eds.), *The development of communication.* New York: Wiley, 1978.

Lucas, E. *Semantic and pragmatic language disorders: Assessment and remediation.* Rockville, MD: Aspen, 1980.

McNeill, D. *The acquisition of language: The study of developmental psycholinguistics.* New York: Harper & Row, 1970.

McShane, J. *Learning to talk.* Cambridge, Eng.: Cambridge University Press, 1980.

Miller, L. Pragmatics: An assessment/intervention model used with an autistic child. Paper presented at the Annual Convention of the American-Speech-Language-Hearing Association, San Francisco, 1978.

Miller, J. *Assessing language production in children.* Baltimore: University Park Press, 1981.

Miller, J., & Yoder, D., A syntax teaching program. In J. McLean, D. Yoder, & R. Schiefelbusch (Eds.), *Language intervention with the retarded.* Baltimore: University Park Press, 1972.

Nelson, K. Structure and strategy in learning to talk. *Monographs of the Society for Research in Child Development,* 1973, *38,* (1-2, Serial No. 149).

Nelson, K.E. Facilitating children's syntax acquisition. *Developmental Psychology,* 1977, *13,* 101-107.

Newhoff, M., Silverman, L., & Millet, A., Linguistic differences in parents' speech to normal and language-disordered children. *Proceedings from the Symposium on Research in Child Language Disorders.* Madison: University of Wisconsin, 1980.

Newport, E., Gleitman, L., & Gleitman, H. I'd rather do it myself. In C. Snow & C. Ferguson, (Eds.), *Talking to children: Language input and acquisition.* Cambridge, Eng.: Cambridge University Press, 1977.

Orazi, D. *A play-oriented approach to early language intervention.* Unpublished master's thesis, Kent State University, 1981.

Pearl, R., Donahue, M., & Bryan, T. Learning-disabled and normal children's responses to requests for clarification which vary in explicitness. Paper presented at the Boston University Conference on Language Development, 1979.

Prizant, B., & Duchan, J. The functions of immediate echolalia in autistic children. *Journal of Speech and Hearing Disorders,* 1981, *46,* 241-249.

128   **Wilcox**

Rees, N. Pragmatics of language: Applications to normal and disordered language development. In R. Sehiefelbusch (Ed.), *Bases of language intervention*. Baltimore: University Park Press, 1978.

Shatz, M., Bernstein, D., & Shulman, M. The responses of language-disordered children to indirect directives in varying contexts, *Applied Psycholinguistics*, 1980, *1*, 295-306.

Snow, C. Mothers' speech to children learning language. *Child Development*, 1972, *43*, 549-565.

Snow, C. The development of conversation between mothers and babies. *Journal of Child Language*, 1977, *4*, 1-22.

Snow, C. Social interaction and language acquisition. In P. Dale & D. Ingram (Eds.), *Child language: An international perspective*. Baltimore: University Park Press, 1981.

Snyder, L. *Pragmatics in language-deficient children: Prelinguistic and early verbal performatives and presuppositions*. Unpublished doctoral dissertation, University of Colorado, 1975.

Stremel, K., & Waryas, C. A behavioral psycholinguistic approach to language training. In L. McReynolds (Ed.), *Developing systematic procedures for training children's language*. American Speech and Hearing Association Monographs, 1974, *18*.

Taenzer, S., Cermak, C., & Hanlon, R. Outside the therapy room: A naturalistic approach to language intervention. *Topics in Learning and Learning Disabilities*, 1981, *1*, 41-46.

Wellman, H., & Lempers, J. The naturalistic communicative abilities of two-year olds. *Child Development*, 1977, *48*, 1052-1057.

Wilcox, M., & Howse, P. Children's use of gestural and verbal behavior in communicative misunderstandings. *Journal of Applied Psycholinguistics*, 1982, *3*, 15-28.

Wilcox, M., & Webster, E. Early discourse behavior: An analysis of children's responses to listener feedback. *Child Development*, 1980, *51*, 1120-1125.

Wilkinson, L., & Rembold, K. The form and function of children's gestures accompanying verbal directives. In P. Dale & D. Ingram (Eds.), *Child language: An international perspective*. Baltimore: University Park Press, 1981.

Lynn S. Snyder, Ph.D.

Developmental Language Disorders: Elementary School Age

When language-disordered children enter elementary school, they seem to disappear. The prevalence of language disorders in preschool children is just above 3% (Leske, 1981). This figure abruptly declines to a figure somewhat closer to 1% in the school-aged population. It would be rewarding to surmise that our programs for the early identification and intervention of language disorders have been so successful that they account for this decline. Unfortunately, as our colleagues working in the schools will tell us, this is not the case.

What, then, is the nature of the great disappearing act that language-disordered children perform when they enter school? To answer this question, we need only look at one other prevalence figure: the prevalence of learning disabilities. It emerges at the elementary school level and ranges between 2% and 8% in the various states (Sheppard, 1981). Careful study of these figures reveals that over time, they changed from 3% to 5% in states like Colorado, where the term "perceptual and communicative disorder" is used in lieu of the term "learning disability." It tends to be lower in states that separate language from learning disabilities.

This great disappearing act is also evident in research. In contrast to the numerous studies of language disorders in preschool children, relatively few studies have been conducted on school-aged children. There are, however, many studies of the language deficits of learning-disabled children.

© College-Hill Press, Inc. All rights, including that of translation, reserved. No part of this publication may be reproduced without the written permission of the publisher.

When language-disordered children enter elementary school, they often come to be associated with different labels: learning-disabled, language- and learning-disabled, reading-disabled, or even dyslexic. It is not that language-disordered children radically change when they reach 6 or 7 years of age. Rather, their problems in processing and producing oral language make it difficult for them to acquire written language: the ability to read, spell, and write composition. In addition, other youngsters are added to their ranks: children who find it difficult to learn written language. Systematic assessment reveals that these children also sustain underlying oral language deficits (Lerner, 1977). It is not surprising that the United States Office of Education defines learning-disabled children as those with intact sensory functioning, normal psychosocial development, general cognitive abilities in the normal range, who demonstrate "a disorder in one or more of the basic psychological processes involved in understanding or using language, spoken or written" (USOE, 1977, p. 65083). This disorder is reflected in a significant discrepancy between age or general abilities and academic achievement. This population, then, seems to constitute the greater proportion of school-aged children with language disorders.

This chapter will examine the semantic, syntactic, morphological, and pragmatic processing and production deficits of these language-disordered youngsters. Since many school-aged children with language disorders have been identified as "learning disabled," or with some similar label, much of the discussion will reference studies of learning-disabled, language- and learning-disabled, reading-disabled, and dyslexic children.

Lexical Processing and Production

The semantic component of language refers to the meaning carried by words. Often our concern with meaning directs our attention to the *lexicon*, or internal dictionary, that one carries in one's head. Although the communicator's internal dictionary is not organized alphabetically like Webster's, it does contain many similar types of information. As Fillmore (1971) pointed out, one's knowledge of a word includes several components. Much like Webster's, it includes information about the phonetic shape of the word, or how it should be pronounced. Like Webster's, it also includes information about the syntactic class to which the word belongs—noun, verb, etc., its primary referential meaning, and any alternate multiple meanings it may carry. The literature suggests that school-aged language-disordered children seem to encounter difficulty processing and producing lexical items.

Word Comprehension

The problems that school-aged language-disordered children encounter with lexical comprehension are not apparent if we look at their ability to comprehend the primary meaning of single words on vocabulary tests such as the *Peabody Picture Vocabulary Test* (PPVT) (Dunn, 1965; Dunn & Dunn, 1981). In fact, studies comparing normal and language/learning-disabled children's comprehension of items on experimental measures (Wiig & Semel, 1973; Wiig, Semel, & Crouse, 1973) indicate that the normal and language/learning-disabled subjects performed similarly on the PPVT. Likewise, Semel and Wiig (1975) found no significant difference between matched normal and language/learning-disabled children's comprehension of vocabulary items on the *Assessment of Children's Language Comprehension* (ACLC) (Foster, Giddan, & Stark, 1973). Rather, school-aged language-disordered children seem to differ from their normal counterparts in their comprehension of specific word categories.

School-aged language/learning-disabled youngsters appear to have particular difficulty comprehending words that express spatial, temporal, and kinship relations. Wiig and Semel (1973) compared the ability of matched normal and language/learning-disabled children to comprehend sentences that employed spatial, temporal, and kinship words, as well as passive constructions and comparative form markers. They found that the language/learning-disabled children performed significantly lower than the normal children on each of these word and form categories. Despite the fact that the youngsters had comparable PPVT scores, they experienced difficulty comprehending the words in these specific categories. If we examine these categories more closely, we find that they are composed of relational words. They do not refer to events, actions, or objects. Rather, these words refer to relationships between objects and/or persons. For example, spatial relationships are often marked by spatial prepositions. Temporal relationships are expressed by the prepositions "before" and "after. " Kinship terms such as "aunt, " "uncle, " and the like relational nouns expressing a familial relationship between two or more persons. These relational words, then, require that the child keep more than one referent in mind. This may be an aspect of lexical processing that is more difficult for language-disordered children.

Word Retrieval

Clinical descriptions of school-aged language/learning-disabled children (DeHirsch, Jansky, & Langford, 1966; Johnson & Myklebust, 1967; Wiig

& Semel, 1976, 1980) have reported that some of these youngsters have difficulty retrieving or accessing words from their lexicon. Typically, these observations have been made while the children were engaged in conversational exchanges. Consequently, it is not always clear whether formulation deficits were also implicated.

In recent years, however, empirical support for these reports has appeared in the literature. Mattis, French, and Rapin's (1975) neuropsy-chological study compared the performance of reading-disabled or dyslexic children, brain-damaged dyslexics, and brain-damaged children with no reading deficits on a variety of cognitive and linguistic measures. They identified three subtypes of disorders that accounted for most of their subjects. The largest subtype demonstrated language deficits. These were characterized by language comprehension problems, syntactic production deficits, poor speech sound discrimination problems, and "anomia," or naming problems. Similarly, Denckla's (1978) retrospective study of dyslexic children seen by her clinic identified three subgroups or subtypes of reading-disabled children. Anomia, or naming problems, was a characteristic attributed to two of the three subgroups that she identified. These studies support the idea that some language/learning-disabled youngsters have word retrieval problems.

More direct tests of these observations can be found in confrontation naming studies which bypass the confounding effects of formulation factors. Denckla (1972) studied the ability of dyslexic, or reading-disabled, boys to name colors and pictured objects. She found that they only experienced color-naming difficulty under rapid and repetitive naming conditions, where they had been instructed to name the colors as quickly as possible. Subsequently, Denckla and Rudel (1976b) examined the rapid automatized naming (RAN) of matched dyslexic, normal, and nondyslexic "low achieving" children between 7 and 12 years of age. Studying the response latencies during the tasks, they found that the dyslexic children were the slowest to respond and name the depicted items, while the normal controls were the fastest. In a similar study, Denckla and Rudel (1976a) compared the performance of dyslexic children, adequate readers with other types of learning problems, and matched normal children between 8 and 11 years of age. All subjects were asked to rapidly name pictured objects. The dyslexic children made more errors than the other groups of children, particularly on low freqeuency words. Error analysis revealed that the majority of the dyslexic children's errors were circumlocutions phonetically similar to the target word. By contrast, the majority of the errors made by the other learning-disabled groups were wrong names that seemed to be visually perceptually based, e.g., a pair of dice was named "Swiss Cheese."

More recently, Wolf (1979) conducted an in-depth study of the word-finding abilities of matched good and poor readers between 6 and 11 years of age. She administered the *Peabody Picture Vocabulary Test;* the *Boston Naming Test;* a picture-naming task in which the stimuli were visually distorted; a rapid automatized naming test for colors, numbers, and letters; phonological (e.g., name as many things as you can that begin with "f") and semantic (e.g., name as many animals as you can) verbal fluency measures; as well as reading tests. She found that the good readers performed significantly better than the poor readers on all naming tests, except the RAN numbers and the visually distorted pictures. The poor readers were particularly deficient in their performance on both measures of verbal fluency. These findings suggest that school-aged learning-disabled children, specifically those with reading deficits, also seem to sustain word-finding problems.

In the same year, German (1979) compared the ability of matched normal and language/learning-disabled children (8 to 11 years of age) on vocabulary comprehension and naming tasks. The groups demonstrated comparable age, general intelligence scores, *Peabody Picture Vocabulary Test* scores, and socioeconomic status. Asking these subjects to name items in pictures, to complete open-ended sentences, and to name objects described, German found that the language/learning-disabled children made significantly more word-finding errors than their matched controls. They found low frequency words in the cloze condition and the naming-to-description condition particularly difficult. Subsequent group analyses revealed that 43% of the learning-disabled children were classified as poor retrievers, performing more than one standard deviation above the mean error rate of the normal children.

Recently, Wiig, Semel, and Nystrom (1982) compared the rapid-naming skills of a group of language/learning-disabled 8- and 9-year-olds with a group of academically achieving 8- and 9-year-olds with normal language development. They assessed the children's ability to rapidly name pictured objects, colors, geometric forms, and colored geometric forms. Their data revealed that the language/learning-disabled children performed significantly worse than their age peers for both time and accuracy when naming pictured objects and colored forms. The total naming time of the language/learning subjects increased as their accuracy decreased. Those language/learning-disabled children who had demonstrated word-finding problems in their spontaneous speech, performed above +1 SD of the mean naming time of the normal group on the object naming measure. These data offer further confirmation of the word-retrieval problems found among school-aged language/learning-disabled children.

Summary

The research of the last decade suggests that many school-aged language-disordered children have lexical processing and production deficits. Although they often demonstrate comparable understanding of single vocabulary words on vocabulary measures, they often have difficulty understanding relational words. Likewise, a number of school-aged language-disordered children have difficulty retrieving words, making more errors in producing names than their normal peers. Thus, selected aspects of the lexicon and the ability to access the words it contains prove difficult for some school-aged language-disordered children.

Syntactic Processing and Production

Some school-aged language-disordered children sustain lexical deficits. In addition, some of these youngsters also seem to have difficulty comprehending and using the syntax and associated morphology of language.

The earlier clinical accounts of DeHirsch et al. (1966) and Johnson and Myklebust (1967) reported that language/learning-disabled children experienced difficulty comprehending and producing syntactic structures. Johnson and Myklebust's anecdotal information suggested a considerable range of severity, with some children sustaining severe deficits. By contrast, the DeHirsch et al. accounts did not reflect this degree of severity. Jansky's later descriptions (1975) characterized the syntactic formulation deficits of language/learning-disabled children as more "subtle." She observed that their spoken language often appears adequate, although it is not really articulate. Sentence formulation is often awkward, characterized by many sentential fragments, simple sentence forms, and the repeated use of stereotypic phrases. Delayed morphological development, particularly in the use of irregular past-tense markers and an over-extended use of pronouns, is also observed. Jansky suggested that these types of problems seem to call less attention to themselves, merely giving one the impression that the child has a less verbal cognitive style. Consequently, these language problems often go unidentified until the children enter school and begin to have problems learning to read and spell. These early observations clearly suggest that language/learning-disabled children may sustain syntactic deficits. Confirmation of these clinical observations came somewhat later with the research of the 70s.

Comprehension of Syntactic and Morphological Forms

One of the earliest tests of the notion that language/learning-disabled children had problems understanding syntactic forms and morphological markers is found in the Wiig and Semel (1973) study discussed earlier. In addition to their comparison of normal and language/learning-disabled children's comprehension of relational terms, they also studied their ability to comprehend passive sentence forms and comparative morphological markers. The language/learning-disabled children also performed significantly worse than their age mates on these items.

More recently, Dixon (1982) compared the ability of 8- and 9-year-old reading-disabled children, age-matched controls, and reading-level controls on several measures of oral language. Despite a number of significant differences between the two groups, she found that the groups were comparable in their comprehension of spoken syntactic and morphological forms. She had assessed their comprehension with the Grammatic Understanding subtest of the *Test of Language Development* (TOLD) (Newcomer & Hammill, 1977). However, this subtest of the TOLD does not seem to adequately sample the syntactic processing that develops during the school years.

Byrne (1981) addressed this question by comparing good and poor second-grade readers' comprehension of late-maturing structures. These included the *John is easy / eager to please* type of constructions identified by Chomsky (1969), and reversible center-embedded, improbable center-embedded, and control relative clause constructions. The *easy / eager to please* constructions were adapted from Cromer (1970), and systematically varied subject, object, and ambiguous adjectives. The following are examples taken from each *easy / eager to please* construction type (Bryne, 1981, p. 206):

Subject-Adjective: *The bird is happy to bite.*

Object-Adjective: *The bird is tasty to bite.*

Ambiguous-Adjective: *The bird is nice to bite.*

Each child was requested to act out the test sentences using hand puppets. Byrne found that while all of the children understood subject-adjective sentence forms equally well, the poor readers tended to assign the logical subjects to the surface structure subject in the object-adjective sentences more frequently than the good readers. Comprehension of the relative clause constructions was assessed by asking the children to point to the one of two pictures that correctly depicted the test sentence. The following are items taken from each of the relative clause construction types as assessed by Byrne (1981, p. 207):

Control sentence: *The fish is biting a yellow frog.*

Reversible sentence: *The cow that the monkey is scaring is yellow.*

Improbable sentence: *The horse that the girl is kicking is brown.*

Again, the poor readers tended to use less mature syntactic processing strategies on these relative clause comprehension tasks. Although both good and poor readers were comparable in their ability to process the reversible clause constructions, the poor readers tended to make more errors on the improbable relative clause sentences. Again, they were more easily seduced into using a less mature syntactic processing strategy. In this case, they used a "probable event" strategy (deVilliers & deVilliers, 1973), in which they ignored the underlying syntactic form and chose the picture depicting the event most likely to occur in the real world. Byrne's data, then, provide nice evidence for the syntactic comprehension deficits sustained by school-aged language/learning-disabled children.

Production of Syntactic and Morphological Forms

Given this evidence for syntactic and morphological processing deficits in language/learning-disabled children, it is not unreasonable to expect that they will also sustain production deficits.

In an early effort to compare the productive language of matched 7 year-old good and poor readers, Fry (1967) and Schulte (1967) subsequently summarized in a paper by Fry, Johnson, and Muehl (1970) exhaustively analyzed oral language samples collected from subjects. They found that the language of the poor readers was characterized by a lower type-token ratio, less frequent use of subject-verb-object frames, and clauses as direct objects, indirect objects, and complements than their normal peers. Transformational analyses revealed that the poor reader's sentences contained fewer transformations than their age mates. Lastly, the poor readers made significantly more errors in subject-verb agreement. Thus, these studies of the syntactic maturity of children with reading problems demonstrate that they often have deficient syntactic formulation.

Recently, Donohue, Pearl, and Bryan (in press) compared the length and syntactic complexity of the sentences produced by matched normal and learning-disabled children. Language samples were collected from the subjects during a classical referential communication task, in which they described figures to an examiner who could not see them. The description of each item would then allow the examiner to select the correct referent from an array set before her. Using the T-unit analysis technique (Golub

& Kidder, 1974; Hunt, 1965), they found that the language/learning-disabled children produced significantly fewer words per T-unit and fewer words per main clause than their normal peers. However, there was no difference in the productivity measures for the two groups. They produced similar numbers of words and T-units. Thus, while the language/ learning-disabled children said as much as their age mates, the syntax of their utterances was not as complex.

A number of studies have examined the ability of language/learning-disabled children to produce appropriate morphological markers. Wiig, Semel, and Crouse's (1973) study of normal, high-risk, and language/ learning-disabled children examined their performance on Berko-Gleason's (1958) measure and the Auditory Association subtest of the *Illinois Test of Psycholinguistic Abilities* (ITPA) (Kirk & McCarthy, 1961). The language/learning-disabled youngsters performed significantly worse than their age mates on both measures of inflectional morphology. Again, the data point to linguistic production deficits in school-aged language/ learning-disabled children.

In a somewhat different study, Vogel (1975, 1977) compared the ability of matched normal and dyslexic second graders on a variety of linguistic and suprasegmental measures. These included a standardized version of Berko-Gleason's (1958) tasks, the *Berry-Talbott Test* (1966), and the Grammatic Closure subtest of the ITPA. She found that the dyslexic children performed significantly worse than their age mates in their ability to morphologically mark real and nonsense words embedded in sentence contexts, as seen in their performance on the ITPA subtest and the Berry-Talbott measures, respectively. These data also corroborate other findings and reports of deficits in the productive morphology of learning-disabled children.

Hook's (1976) study explored the inflectional morphology of matched normal and learning-disabled fourth-grade children. Using the same measures as Vogel, she replicated Vogel's findings in this older age group.

Subsequently, Moran and Byrne (1977) explored one aspect of inflectional morphology—verb-tense markers—in greater depth. Noting Leonard's (1972) observation that the inappropriate use of verb forms has often characterized deviant language skills, they systematically compared the ability of matched groups of normal and language/learning-disabled children to produce appropriate verb-tense markers. They sampled their subjects' ability to produce three regular past-tense verbs formed by adding /-d, /-t, and /-əd/. In addition, they also examined the formation of seven irregular verb categories based upon Greenbaum, Quirk, Leach, and Svartnik's (1972) classification system. Analysis of their data revealed that the language/learning-disabled children made significantly more errors across all ten categories. In addition, it appeared that they used qualitatively different strategies for marking past tense. For example, they often avoided using past-tense markers by frequent use of the form "did" with an uninflected form of the verb—"she did climb." In addition, the language/learning-disabled children were three times more likely than their normal age mates to produce an uninflected root verb than a past-tense marker. They were also more likely to use redundant markers than their normal peers, e.g., "jumpted." Thus, their inflectional morphology was not only significantly different from that of normal children, it also appeared to be somewhat deviant.

Dixon's (1982) comparison of age-matched, reading-level matched, and reading-disabled 8- and 9-year-olds also included a measure of productive inflectional morphology. She found that the reading-disabled group performed significantly worse than both their age-matched and reading-level matched controls. Clearly, the early clinical observations of Johnson and Myklebust (1967) and DeHirsch et al. (1966) that noted the language/learning-disabled child's difficulty marking word inflections have been well supported by empirical studies.

If these youngsters are deficient in their productive syntax and morphology, it might be interesting to know whether they can recognize and/or correct ungrammatical productions. Liles, Schulman, and Bartlett (1977) compared the ability of normal and language-disabled 5- to 7-year-olds to make judgments of grammaticality, and to correct ungrammatical sentences. They found that the language-disabled youngsters attempted to correct only 78% of the agrammatical sentences in contrast to 97% attempted by their controls. Further, approximately 90% of the corrections made by the controls in each error category—syntactic agreement, lexical violation, and word order—were correct. By contrast, the language-disordered children were able to correctly revise only 21% of the sentences assessing syntactic agreement, 42% of the lexical violations, and 41% of the word-order errors. These data suggest that school-aged language-disordered children have difficulty recognizing syntactic errors when they occur and knowing how to revise them acceptably. In light of earlier evidence for syntactic production deficits in school-aged language-disordered children, these results are not unreasonable.

Summary
School-aged language/learning-disabled children seem to have difficulty processing and producing syntactic and morphological forms, and they seem to be late at learning those underlying syntactic structures that develop

during the elementary school years. Similarly, the transformational complexity of their productive output is also reduced. They also seem to have difficulty producing appropriate irregular morphological forms and handling syntactic agreement. Thus, even during the elementary school years, language/learning-disabled children have difficulty with the syntactic component of language.

Pragmatic Processing and Production

With the publication of Bates' *Language and Context,* (1976), basic and applied psycholinguistic research took a new direction. Our post-Chomskian fascination with children's developing comprehension and production of syntactic forms gave way to a concern with how these forms were mobilized to achieve communicative goals. Observers of normal and disordered child language studied the functions of the child's utterances or the uses to which they were put, in addition to the syntactic forms they assumed. Thus, they looked at the types of speech acts children performed with their utterances. These included direct and indirect requests or directives (Ervin-Tripp, 1977), acknowledgments, solicitations, responses, and threats (Dore, 1978). It became apparent that by the time children entered elementary school, they comprehended and had productive control over many direct and indirect ways of requesting things, acknowledging and answering others, and achieving a variety of social goals (Ervin-Tripp, 1977).

It also became obvious that children not only could accomplish these pragmatic or functional goals on the utterance level, but could amortize their requesting strategies across conversational turns (Ervin-Tripp, 1977). Thus, they gradually "set up" their listener during the course of the conversation. In addition, they learned to initiate, develop, and maintain conversational topics, structure their discourse narrative, and revise their utterances (Gallagher, 1977). Similarly, they were increasingly able to process larger units of narrative discourse and acquired the ability to draw inferences between utterances in discourse (Johnson & Smith, 1981; Stein & Glenn, 1979).

Just as language/learning-disabled children experience difficulty with the structural aspects of language, they often find it difficult to handle the functional or pragmatic aspects of the system.

Processing Pragmatic Structures

The psycholinguistic study of the pragmatic aspects of language has suggested some underlying functional organization to language in addition to its structural organization (Bates, 1976; Clark & Haviland, 1977; Green-field & Smith, 1976; Kintsch, 1974, 1977). Individuals are able to go beyond identification of the syntactic frame to understand the speaker's underlying intention. Children learn to do this as well. They come to realize that one communicative intention can be expressed with many different syntactic forms. Conversely, they also learn that one syntactic form can express many different communicative intentions.

Sentences also seem to have a specific functional organization. The topic of a conversational point is systematically identified by a variety of syntactic and lexical devices. In English, it is usually expressed by the subject of a sentence. Once the topic has been identified or named, the conversational partners consider it "given" information. They then make comments or share "new" information about it (Haviland & Clark, 1974). This topic/comment organization of language occurs at both the sentence and the discourse, or conversational, level. At the sentence level, speakers identify their topic and comment about it. In discourse, they identify main topics and subtopics, often nesting subtopics within the main topics. They make comments that are related to those topics or subtopics (Bates & Mac-Whinney, in press). Using syntactic devices to mark new topics, they direct the flow of conversation from one topic to another.

Individuals seem to expect speakers to adhere to this functional organization of topic ("given" information) and comment ("new" information). Clark and Haviland (1977) suggest that, in a sense, conversational partners have a given-new contract. The speaker assumes that the listener knows a particular piece, or pieces, of information. This "given" information forms the topic for the comment, or " new, " information the speaker wishes to share. His listener locates the given information in the utterance and searches his memory for this piece of world knowledge. He then attaches the new information to it. Thus, conversational speakers must consider or estimate the "given" information—the prior knowledge, beliefs, assumptions, and experiences—they share with their listeners. In this way, they keep the given-new contract and insure effective communication.

Speakers and listeners seem to adhere to the given-new contract on both the sentence and discourse level. At the sentence level, speakers use syntactic and lexical devices to signal given and new information. Their listeners use their own linguistic knowledge of these devices to isolate given and new pieces of information.

On the discourse level, the "given" part of the contract can take on interesting charcteristics. A speaker may assume that a listener has some knowledge of events, such as going to a movie or a bank. He assumes that the listener has organized the basic information contained in those events in a way similar to his own. Consequently, they share the same "script"

(Schank & Abelson, 1977) for the event. For example, they both know that one purchases a ticket for the movie, gives it to the usher, is admitted, enters the theater area, seats oneself, views the film, and leaves. While each may have some different specific scripts, e.g., for drive-in movies or for a subscription series at the art museum, they share a generic script that organizes the component events and identifies the roles assumed by the participants. Scriptal information seems to facilitate comprehension of longer units of discourse, particularly narrative discourse or stories (Rumelhardt, 1980). The listener activates his script for the event that has been given. He then attaches the pieces of new information contained in the narrative to the component events and roles of the script that he has activated (Anderson, Spiro, & Anderson, 1978). The listener and reader have scripts for stories, as well as for events. These are often referred to as story schemata (Kintsch, 1974) or story grammars (Mandler & Johnson, 1978; Stein & Glenn, 1979). These types of structures seem to organize and facilitate the comprehension of discourse narratives (Kintsch & Kintsch, 1979).

Lastly, when speakers fail to indentify a "given" referent clearly or consistently, listeners use their scripts to draw inferences. They use their scripts to construct information the speaker has not explicitly stated (Haviland & Clark, 1974; Kintsch, 1974, 1977). For example, referring to Mary as "she" in a sentence during a new subtopic forces the listener to draw an inference that "she" refers to the woman, Mary, who was discussed several sentences earlier. Or, take the following sentences used by Clark and Haviland (1974): *Horace got some picnic supplies out of the trunk. The beer was warm.* It was never explicitly stated that Horace had packed beer. However, listeners seem to activate their "picnic" scripts, which suggest that picnic supplies often include beer. Thus, they infer that Horace had included beer in his picnic supplies (Haviland & Clark, 1974).

Listeners seem to engage in many types of functional or pragmatically based operations as they process sentence and discourse level information.

Sentence Level Processes

At face value, it seems that it must be difficult to figure out a speaker's underlying intention even when it differs from the syntactic form of the sentence. Children, however, seem to master this skill during their preschool years (Shatz, 1978). In an early effort to determine whether 5- to 7-year-old language-disordered children can comprehend indirect speech acts, Prinz (1977; in press) compared their ability to comprehend direct and indirect requests with younger normal children at comparable language levels.

He found that the language-disordered children did not differ significantly from the normal children with whom they had been matched.

Other pragmatic structures processed at the sentence level included identification of given and new information. This has been explored recently in learning-disabled youngsters. Donohue (1981a), using Hornby's (1971) experimental paradigm, compared the ability of matched normal and learning-disabled children to comprehend and use syntactic devices that indicated given vs. new information. At this point, the discussion will be confined to the comprehension phase of the experiment. Specifically, she asked each child to listen to sentences, and indicate which of two pictures was described. The sentences took one of five syntactic forms, and described an actor-action-object relationship. However, since the test sentences did not accurately describe either of the pictures, the child's answer indicated the sentential component that he regarded as the given information. Although Donohue observed the expected developmental and sentence-type effects, she found no significant differences between the performance of the normal and learning-disabled children.

At this point, the available literature suggests that school-aged language-disordered children seem to process sentence-level pragmatic structures as well as their peers. They can comprehend a variety of indirect requests. In addition, they seem to be able to understand the various syntactic devices used to signal given vs. new information.

Discourse Level Processes: Conversation

Although school-aged language-disordered children seem to have mastered pragmatic processing at the sentence level, this does not seem to hold true at the level of discourse. This can be seen in a study of their ability to understand conversational rules, as well as in a number of studies of their narrative discourse processing.

Comparing the conversational skills of matched normal and learning-disabled school children, Donohue, Pearl, and Bryan (1980) studied their ability to request clarification of messages based on the informational adequacy of the message. Using the classic referential paradigm of screened interlocutors, Donohue et al. asked each child to identify a drawing from a plate containing four choices. The child was instructed by one examiner that his "partner" behind the screen could give him clues which would help him choose the correct picture. If he was not sure which drawing was the correct choice, he could ask her questions. This examiner also ran trial items with the child to insure that he understood the task, as well as the opportunity to query the speaker. His "partner," a second examiner, entered, sat behind the screen, and described each item to the child. The messages differed in the amount of information the child needed to correctly identify the picture, being either fully informative, partially informative, or uninformative. The first examiner was present on the child's side of the screen, recording the child's responses. Subsequently, the child was asked to judge messages given by other people. The child had to indicate whether the message would allow a listener to choose the correct drawing.

Analysis of the subjects' responses to the communication task revealed several significant differences. First, there were clear developmental effects in children's ability to realize when they were given inadequate clues. Older children were more likely to recognize less-adequate messages, request clarification, and, thus, choose the correct drawing. The learning-disabled children did not differ from the normal children in their ability to use the informative messages to select a correct picture. However, they were less likely to request clarification of the less-informative messages. Consequently, they had greater difficulty than their age mates in making the correct choices from the less-informative clues. Analysis of the children's performance on the appraisal task revealed that most of the learning-disabled children were able to *recognize* less-adequate messages. Analyses of request forms they produced indicated that they had the necessary linguistic skill to request clarification of messages. Despite these abilities, they made fewer requests for clarification. Donohue et al. suggest that they failed to understand their role as a conversational listener. The learning-disabled subjects did not seem to realize that, as listeners, they were obligated to let the speaker know when a message was unclear. These findings, then, suggest that some aspects of processing conversational discourse pose problems for the school-aged language/learning-disabled child.

Discourse Level Processes: Narratives

In addition to processing conversation, individuals also process discourse narratives or stories they hear. Professionals, using an educational model, have traditionally referred to this as listening comprehension (Durrell, 1965). Others, (e.g., Graybeal, 1981) refer to it as memory. Cognitive and experimental psychologists (Freedle, 1977; Just & Carpenter, 1977; Kintsch, 1974, 1977; Rumelhardt, 1980) have typically considered it discourse comprehension. Using a variety of recognition, verification, and recall experiments, the cognitive psychologists cited above and their colleagues have observed that individuals seem to understand discourse in terms of their schemata or knowledge of scripts, narratives, and other aspects of the world (Rumelhardt, 1980).

Individuals make such strong use of this strategy that when a narrative contains information that does not match the listener's, they understand the story only in terms of their own schemata—thus, "misunderstanding" the story. For example, in his now-classic experiment, Bartlett (1932) asked subjects to listen to an American Indian story. The narrative schema, or story structure, of the Indian myth was quite different from the structure of Western European narratives. When his subjects retold it, their versions did not resemble the original story. What they had done was to interpret the Indian tale in terms of the Western European tale "script" they knew so well. They changed the Indian tale to conform to their own story scripts! These results were recently replicated in a study by Kintsch and Green (1978), where subjects were presented with schema-conforming stories and Alaskan Indian myths. Anderson, Spiro, and Anderson (1978) suggest that these scripts or schemata are "ideational scaffolding." The listener takes in information, activates the schema or generic script that matches it, and anchors to it the information in the narrative. Thus, the listener understands the new information presented to him in relation to his existing knowledge.

The ability to process units as large as narrative discourse or stories develops during middle childhood. The amount of information children can understand and recall from stories increases as a function of age (Christie & Schumacher, 1975; Mandler & Johnson, 1977; Stein & Glenn, 1979). This developmental trend continues throughout the elementary school years (Stein & Glenn, 1979). School-aged children seem to remember story settings, beginnings, and outcomes best (Mandler & Johnson, 1977; Stein & Glenn, 1979). As they mature, they seem to acquire improved recall for the main characters' internal reactions and outcomes.

Many language/learning-disabled children seem to have difficulty with this type of processing. Have you ever tried to get them to tell you about a recent movie or television show they have seen?

A study of the discourse-processing of normal and reading-disabled children conducted by Weaver and Dickenson (1979) also included reading Stein and Glenn's (1979) stories to the children and asking the dyslexic subjects to recall the narratives. They compared their performance to that of Stein and Glenn's sample. Examining the number of ideas recalled, they found no significant differences between the two groups. However, their reading-disabled children included those with both high and low verbal abilities. When Weaver and Dickenson conducted a within-group analysis of the performance of their reading-disabled subjects, they found that the poor readers with high verbal ability recalled significantly more ideas than those with low verbal ability. These data lend further support for the presence of discourse-processing deficits in *some* reading-disabled youngsters.

In a similar study, Graybeal (1981) compared the ability of matched school-aged normal and language-impaired children to recall stories read to them. She tested each language-impaired child to determine that she or he possessed the vocabulary and syntactic comprehension skills needed to process the stories. Each child listened to and was asked to recall two stories, structured after Mandler and Johnson's (1977) story grammar. She found that the normal children recalled significantly more information than the language-impaired children. Again, the available evidence suggests that language-disordered children sustain discourse-processing deficits.

One might argue, however, that the language/learning-disabled children described here performed poorly because they may have had productive-language deficits. All of these studies asked subjects to retell the stories. If—as we know—language/learning-disabled children also have productive-language deficits, then these deficits might limit the amount of information they produce during recall. Snyder, Haas, and Becker (1982) investigated this question, asking normal and language/learning-disabled children probe-recall questions after they had retold a story. Once again, the normal children recalled significantly more information than the learning-disabled. And, they continued to recall more information during probe-recall questions that required little productive language. Thus, school-aged language/learning-disabled children seem to sustain true deficits in discourse-processing which do not seem to be related to the confounding effect of productive language deficits.

Discourse Level Processes: Inferences

The work of Clark and Haviland (1977), Keenan and Kintsch (1974), Trabasso and Nicholas (1977), and others have clearly demonstrated that listeners go beyond the information that is explicitly contained in the message. Using their schemata, or scripted knowledge, and the assumptions they share with the speakers, they interpret messages and construct meanings that were never explicitly stated. They draw inferences such as the types described earlier as well as a variety of others (Trabasso & Nicholas, 1977).

Young children acquire the ability to draw inferences. They develop the ability to answer questions about implied information (Kail, Chi, Ingram, & Danner, 1977; Paris & Upton, 1976), to make transitive inferences when they have encoded the premises (Riley & Trabasso, 1974; Trabasso, 1975), and to infer antecedent states and causes and predict outcomes in situations with familiar scripts (Gelman, Bullock, & Meck, 1980). In addition to these "local" inferences, they also acquire the ability to make "global" inferences, which draw upon information that has occurred in previous episodes or scenes in the story (Johnson & Smith, 1981).

Just as learning-disabled youngsters have difficulty mobilizing their schemata for story comprehension, they also have difficulty mobilizing them to draw inferences. In the previously cited study by Weaver and Dickenson (1979), they found that the reading-disabled children made significantly fewer minor inferences than normally developing children.

Ellis-Weismer (1981) compared the inferential skills of school-aged language-disordered children to one group of normal children with comparable nonverbal cognitive abilities, and another group of normal children at a similar level of language comprehension. Specifically, she examined their ability to draw spatial and causal inferences from short narratives presented in two ways: verbally and pictorially. She found that under both conditions, the language-disordered children performed like the normal children with similar comprehension skills. The normal children with similar nonverbal cognitive abilities performed significantly better than these two groups in the verbal condition for both explicitly stated information and information that had to be inferred. On the pictorial condition, they performed better only on the inferential items. These findings seem to offer support for the notion that language-disordered children sustain deficits in their inferential abilities.

Lastly, the Snyder et al. (1982) study cited earlier also investigated the ability of language/learning-disabled sixth-grade children to draw inferences. Using a probe-question paradigm, they assessed their subjects' ability to draw a variety of inferences: spatial, causal, world knowledge, and social motivational. Overall, they found that the language/learning-disabled were less proficient at drawing inferences than their age mates.

These studies provide some baseline indices that language/learning-disabled children may sustain a variety of discourse processing deficits.

Producing Pragmatic Structures

Pragmatic competence typically includes the ability to produce—as well as process—the various pragmatic structures. This includes the production of a wide variety of speech acts, particularly formulation of indirect forms. It also includes the ability to revise one's utterances in response to the needs of the listener. And, it goes beyond the sentence level to the production of effective conversations. Recent research has begun to focus on the ability of school-aged language-disordered children to produce pragmatic structures.

Producing Pragmatic Structures: Sentence level

Young children can produce a wide variety of speech acts by the time they enter elementary school. This is not necessarily true, however, of language-disordered children. Prinz (1977) compared the performance of young normal children matched with language-impaired children for linguistic level. In a free-play situation, he found that the language-disordered children used fewer declarative hints and more interrogatives to request actions and objects than the younger normal children. In an experimental situation in which its subjects requested things from a hand puppet, Prinz found that the language disordered children used fewer formal linguistic devices, e.g., contrastive stress, conditional mood, and so forth, to signal polite requests.

In a subsequent study, Prinz (in press) studied the requesting strategies of language-disordered children from 3½ to 8 years of age. During the free-play condition in this study, he made a "doctor" kit available to the children. Prinz found that, in this situation, the proportion of indirect requests produced by the language-disordered children decreased as a function of age. This observation is at variance with the literature on the normal development of request forms (Ervin-Tripp, 1977; Garvey, 1975). His findings, however, may be related to the use of the "doctor" kit. Research on requests produced during role-playing in this situation (Andersen, 1977, 1978) has revealed that high proportions of direct requests are associated with these types of roles. Thus, the increased proportion of direct requests produced by the older language-disordered children may have reflected their growing awareness of the sociolinguistic aspects of role-playing.

Prinz's findings are somewhat difficult to judge. His initial study observed distinct deficits in the requesting behavior of language-disordered children. His subsequent study revealed developmental trends similar to those observed in normal children. Since the latter study was a single-group investigation, it is difficult to know whether the requests produced by his language-disordered subjects were deficient, despite the developmental effects observed.

More recently, Donohue (1981b) compared the requesting strategies of matched normal and learning-disabled children. Asking the children to request a newspaper from imaginary listeners with rather different power and familiarity characteristics, she analyzed the politeness of their requests and the nature of their appeals. She found that the two groups did not differ in the variety of request forms produced. Interestingly, the learning-disabled girls were more polite to all listeners. When the children's responses to the power vs. intimacy dimensions of their listeners were examined, Donohue found that the normal boys were more polite to nonintimate listeners, while the learning-disabled boys were more polite to low-power or low-dominance listeners. Thus, the learning disabled boys did differ in the politeness of their request, but they did not understand the conversational implications of the intimacy and power of the listener. In that these learning-disabled boys were able to vary their request forms, Donohue has interpreted this as evidence for a deficit in social cognition.

Producing Pragmatic Structures: Conversation

An important aspect of conversational competence is the ability to communicate new information to a listener effectively. In an early effort to study this skill, Meline (1978) compared school-aged language-disordered children with younger normal children who had similar levels of productive language development. Using the screened-listener paradigm, he asked each child to direct an adult listener in placing blocks into a pattern that matched the child's pattern. When one judged communicative effectiveness in terms of whether the listener chose the correct referent, the language-disordered children performed more successfully than their language-matched controls. However, when one compared the children in terms of the proportion of communicatively effective responses to the quantity of verbal output, the group differences disappeared. Preliminary data on a group of normal age peers revealed that they performed better than the language-disordered children. Thus, the language-disordered children in his study were not as communicatively effective as their more linguistically advanced age mates. Yet, they performed better than younger, linguistically similar children. They seemed to achieve this communicative success by saying more to their listener.

Perhaps one of the more challenging pragmatic tasks for an individual is engaging a listener in conversation, particularly a noncompliant, or socially powerful, listener, and achieving one's social goals with that person. This task might not be so tricky if listeners did not behave so unpredictably. Despite its difficulty, normal children seem to acquire the skill gradually, becoming remarkably proficient by adolescence. This is not so true of language/learning-disabled children.

In a rather interesting study of normal and learning-disabled children, Bryan, Donohue, and Pearl (1981) examined their conversational persuasion skills. Each child and two of his classmates were asked to rank-order gift choices for their class. Each subject was then taken aside. Half of the subjects in each group were given a "pep talk," and told that they had made good choices and should convince the others to make the same choices. The other half of the subjects were simply told "okay" and directed to the testing location. Analysis of the findings revealed that the learning-disabled children were less conversationally persuasive than their normal peers. The "pep talk" did not have any effect on their efforts. The learning-disabled children appeared to be more conversationally compliant than their peers. In addition, they did less to regulate or direct the flow of the conversation, making fewer attempts to monitor the conversation and fewer bids to hold the conversational floor. Thus, the learning-disabled children appeared to be less dominant, less assertive, and more compliant conversational partners.

In another attempt to examine learning-disabled children's ability to regulate and direct a conversation, Bryan, Donohue, Pearl, and Sturm (1981) studied their conversational skills when they were placed in a dominant role. They compared the conversational skills of matched normal and learning-disabled second- and fourth-grade children. Each child was placed into a pretend "TV Talk Show" situation where she or he was cast as the show's host. An academically achieving classmate was cast as the "talk show guest." Analysis of the children's conversations revealed that the learning-disabled children and their normal controls participated with the same frequency in the conversation, taking a similar number of conversational turns. In general, the learning-disabled children asked fewer questions. Specifically, they asked fewer open-ended questions than the normal children. Consequently, their "guests" were less likely to provide elaborated answers to questions, and in fact, they tended to ask their learning-disabled "hosts" more single-response questions. Not surprisingly, more role switching occurred when the learning-disabled children were "hosts" than when the nondisabled children assumed that dominant role. Despite the fact that this situational context clearly placed learning-disabled children in the socially dominant role, they were less able to benefit from this conversational advantage than their peers. Even when the "deck is loaded" in their favor, learning-disabled children continue to be more deferential and less assertive conversational partners.

In general, language/learning-disabled children seem to be less assertive conversational partners and to have difficulty understanding their role and all that it entails.

Summary

Although elementary school-age language/learning-disabled children seem to comprehend a wide variety of indirect and direct speech acts, they appear to have problems producing indirect forms. They also seem to have difficulty processing and producing the pragmatic aspects of discourse. They find aspects of both conversational and narrative discourse problematic and their comprehension of narrative discourse does not seem as complete or as organized as their age mates. As conversational partners, language/learning-disabled children seem to be more passive and agreeable partners, who cannot control the flow of conversation even when its direction is their responsibility. Thus, school-aged language-disordered children appear to have significant problems handling the pragmatic aspects of language.

Specific Cognitive Deficits

Both language-disordered children and learning-disabled children are characterized by their intact general cognitive abilities. Their language deficits, therefore, are not related to some form of mental retardation. In fact, the disorder is defined in terms of the discrepancy between the child's linguistic skills—oral and/or written—and general cognitive abilities. A few recent studies, however, have suggested that such a child may sustain impairment or delayed maturation of one specific cognitive skill— anticipatory imagery. *Anticipatory imagery* refers to the ability to look at an object or form, represent it mentally, and be able to rotate the mental visual symbol so that its position in space after several successive rotations can be anticipated (Piaget & Inhelder, 1971). This skill is typically assessed with spatial rotation tasks such as the higher level items of the *Ayres Space Test* and the *Minnesota Paper Form Board.* On the *Ayres Space Test,* for example, in the higher level items a puzzle form and two puzzle pieces are placed before the child, with the pieces partially rotated. Only one piece actually fits the puzzle. The child must determine—without touching or manipulating the stimuli—the piece that will actually complete the puzzle. In contrast to the static imagery of visual discrimination and visual-closure tasks, anticipatory imagery is considered dynamic and highly representational.

Recent interest in this ability of school-aged language-disordered youngsters was sparked by Johnston and Ramstad's (1977) study. Motivated by aspects of the relationship between language and cognition, they administered a series of classical Piagetian tasks to language-impaired preadolescents between 10 and 12 years of age. Their initial analyses revealed that all but one of their subjects had not reached the concrete operational stage level of performance on more than half of the tasks in their battery. In a subsequent task analysis, they separated their tasks into those that had required the processing of more complex verbal stimuli vs. those that had required the ablity to anticipate transformed physical states. Johnston and Ramstad found that all of their subjects experienced greatest difficulty on those tasks requiring anticipatory imagery. By contrast, they had the least difficulty on those tasks using complex verbal stimuli. This was a rather startling result for *language*-disordered children! They concluded that their language-disordered subjects' concomitant delays in anticipatory imagery might be related to a more basic deficit in the ability to mobilize symbols.

Subsequently, Murphy (1978) and Murphy and Stephens (in preparation) sought to compare the anticipatory imagery of normal and language-disordered children between 5 and 8½ years of age. Their subjects were matched for chronological age and performance on the *Raven's Coloured Progressive Matrices*. The language-disordered youngsters, however, did not seem to demonstrate particularly significant impairment. Ten of their eleven subjects scored *at* or just below the *28th* percentile, with one scoring at the 60th percentile on the Developmental Sentence Scoring (DSS). Such scores seem to represent the low end of the normal range. On a language-screening measure, only eight subjects failed the syntactic screening. Murphy and Stephens administered a series of Piagetian anticipatory imagery tasks and psychometric spatial tasks requiring anticipatory imagery. They found no significant differences between the two groups. These results are not surprising. First, they matched their groups on performance on the Ravens Matrices, a task which requires some anticipatory imagery at some levels. Second, a number of their "language-disordered" subjects did not appear to demonstrate a *significant* discrepancy between productive language abilities and general cognitive abilities. For the *most part*, they seem to have been comparing high verbal and low verbal *normal* children.

Another test of these notions was in a study by Savich (1980). She compared the ability of age-matched normal and language-disordered children between 7½ and 9½ years of age. The language-disordered children demonstrated language performance beyond one standard deviation below the mean on a standardized measure. They also demonstrated general cognitive abilities within the normal range. Savich assessed her subjects' visual analytic and visual gestaltist abilities, as well as their anticipatory imagery, using Piagetian and psychometric measures. Her findings indicated that the language-disordered children were far less accurate on all tasks requiring anticipation of the transformation of visual state or mental rotation, as well as on the visual analytic task. By contrast, they performed as well as their peers on one of the two gestaltist measures. Savich felt that these findings supported the specific cognitive deficit hypothesis: the ability to represent or symbolize information, and transform the symbolic representation a number of times, regardless of sensory channel—auditory/vocal or visual—is deficient in school-aged language-disordered children.

These studies provide some recent support for the link between specific cognitive abilities and language development. The results of the Johnston and Ramstad (1977) and Savich (1980) studies suggest that anticipatory imagery—that cognitive ability which makes its greatest developmental strides from 7 to 11 years of age—is deficient in school-aged language-disordered youngsters. Interestingly, Khami's (1981) comparative study of normal and language-disordered preschoolers demonstrated no significant group differences for one traditional test of anticipatory imagery, mental displacement, and differences for another test—haptic recognition. Although Khami interpreted the language-disordered children's deficient haptic recognition as evidence of deficits in anticipatory imagery, it is interesting to note they were similar to their normal counterparts on the more traditional measure of anticipatory imagery. Examining the distribution of his scores, it appears that all of his subjects were still at the early levels of skill development for that task. This skill is not expected to make its greatest gains for another 2 to 3 years. Consequently, one would not expect differences to emerge until that time.

Regardless of the differences between Khami's (1981) interpretation of his results and the interpretation put forward here, the critical point is the observed deficit in mental rotation or anticipatory imagery skills of language-disordered children. Since Strauss and Lehtinen (1947), we have alluded to the concomitant visual perceptual deficits of language-disordered and learning-disabled children. These findings suggest that they may not sustain deficits at the level of visual feature analysis. Rather, the "visual perceptual" deficits that we observe may be symptomatic of underlying representational, or even sequential, analytic deficits.

Recent Advances and an Age-Old Dilemma: Identification and Assessment of School-Aged Language-Disordered Children

Significant Discrepancy

The growing interest of our consumers, and our corresponding need for accountability, as well as the increased rigor demanded by our own research, have mandated that clinicians demonstrate that language-disordered youngsters' communicative skills are significantly discrepant from their general cognitive abilities. Translated operationally, this means that they should perform beyond -1 standard deviation below the mean, plus the test's standard error of measurement. The mean, however, is the mean projected given the child's general cognitive abilities. In some instances the term "general cognitive abilities" is interpreted as the child's nonverbal IQ. In other instances it is interpreted as his full scale IQ.

While this appears to be a rather straightforward standard, it is difficult to implement, particularly with school-aged children. First, a number of our existing diagnostic tools fail to report the standard error of measurement, or figures from which it might be derived. Second, we lack a sufficient number of standardized measures that extend beyond 8 years of age.

Only recently, have a few measures emerged that can be used with youngsters older than 8 years. These include Wiig and Semel's (1981) *Clinical Evaluation of Language Function* (CELF); *The Word Test* (Jorgensen, Barrett, Huisingh, and Zachman, 1981); and Gardner's *One Word Expressive Vocabulary Test* (1980). Third, none of the syntactic and pragmatic processing and production abilities thought to emerge during the elementary school years are sampled by our existing diagnostic measures of language development. Understandably, we need not apologize for our failure to do this in the pragmatic domain. Sufficient basic information has yet to be developed for normal children. However, we can hardly make this claim relative to the syntactic domain. Carol Chomsky's work emerged in 1969, followed closely by Kessel's (1970). More than a decade has passed since this research was conducted. Fourth, the problem is compounded by our lack of consensus regarding what constitutes a significant discrepancy in language development. Do we agree with Stark and Tallal's (1981) criteria, which suggest that the child must demonstrate both a receptive *and* expressive deficit? Or, can we include the group of youngsters whom they had observed exhibiting deficits in expressive skills alone? Similarly, how shall we regard the language/learning-disabled child? Is this a "mixed disorder" (Stark & Tallal, 1981)?

Thus, despite our new knowledge, it remains difficult to adequately identify and assess school-aged children with significant discrepancies in their oral language development.

The Territorial Imperative

The great disappearing act performed by elementary-school language-disordered children raises an uncomfortable issue: territorial rights. If we consider the logistics and administrative demands to report the number of children who receive special services, it becomes important to identify those children needing language intervention. Our ability to identify the underlying oral-language deficits of "learning-disabled" youngsters has been limited by the paucity of appropriate measures of syntactic development. Consequently, many of these youngsters are seen by special educators who focus their efforts on the children's visual-perceptual, visual-motor, and written-language skills. Current research, however, suggests that the majority of these youngsters sustain underlying oral-language deficits. If more viable measures of the syntactic development of school-aged children were available, some of them might be identified for language-intervention programming. Surely, a combined approach might prove more effective for these children.

One wonders, however, if we are afraid to assert our territorial rights.

Or, are we afraid to infringe upon the territorial claims of other professions—despite the mounting evidence for underlying oral language deficits in "learning" disabled children?

Conclusion

Current research suggests that language-disordered children of elementary school age sustain significant deficits in the processing and production of oral language. Unfortunately, our ability to identify and document these deficits beyond the experimental setting has been limited. Consequently, our charge seems clear. We need to translate our empirically derived knowledge of the normal and disordered language development of elementary-school children into tools for clinical assessment. Admittedly, this is not an easy task, but we would hope that some of our colleagues will rise to the challenge.

References

Andersen, E. Young children's knowledge of role-related speech differences: A mommy is not a daddy is not a baby. *Papers and Reports in Child Language Development*, 1977, *13*, 91-98.

Andersen, E. Will you don't snore please? Directives in young children's role-play speech. *Papers and Reports in Child Language Development*, 1978, *15*, 140-160.

Anderson, R. C., Spiro, R. J., & Anderson, M.C. Schemata as scaffolding for the representation of information in connected discourse. *American Educational Research Journal*, 1978, *15*, 433-440.

Bartlett, F.C. *Remembering*. Cambridge, Eng: Cambridge University Press, 1932.

Bates, E. *Language and context: Studies in the acquisition of pragmatics*. New York: Academic Press, 1976.

Bates, E., & MacWhinney, B. Functionalist approaches to grammar. In L. Gleitman & E. Wanner (Eds.), *Language acquisition: The state of the art*. New York: Cambridge University Press, in press.

Berko, J. The child's learning of English morphology. *Word*, 1958, *14*, 75-96.

Berry, M., & Talbott, S. *Berry-Talbott Language Tests, 1: Comprehension of Grammar*. Rockford, IL. 1966.

Bryan, T., Donohue, M., & Pearl, R. Learning disabled children's peer interactions during a small group problem solving task. *Learning Disability Quarterly*, 1981, *4*, 13-22.

Bryan, T., Donohue, M., Pearl, R., & Sturm, C. Learning disabled children's conversational skills: The "TV Talk Show." *Learning Disability Quarterly*, 1981, *4*, 250-259.

Byrne, B. Deficient syntactic control in poor readers: Is a weak phonetic memory code responsible? *Applied Psycholinguistics*, 1981, *2*, 201-212.

Chomsky, C.S. *The acquisition of syntax in children from 5 to 10*. Cambridge, Mass: MIT Press, 1969.

Christie, D.J., & Schumacher, G.M. Developmental trends in the abstraction and recall of relevant versus irrelevant thematic information from connected verbal materials. *Child Development*, 1975, *46*, 598-602.

Clark, H.H., & Haviland, S.E. Comprehension and the given-new contract. In R.O. Freedle (Ed.), *Discourse production and comprehension* (Vol. 1) Norwood, NJ: Ablex, 1977.

Cromer, R.F. "Children are nice to understand": Surface structure clues for the recovery of a deep structure. *British Journal of Psychology*, 1970, *61*, 397-408.

De Hirsch, K., Jansky, J., & Langford, W.S. *Predicting reading failures*. New York: Harper & Row, 1966.

Denckla, M.B. Color-naming defects in dyslexic boys. *Cortex*, 1972, *8*, 164-176.

Denckla, M.B. Retrospective study and dyslexic children (1975). Reported in A.L. Benton & D. Pearl (Eds.), *Dyslexia: An appraisal of current knowledge*. New York: Oxford University Press, 1978.

Denckla, M.B., & Rudel, R. Naming of object drawings by dyslexic and other learning disabled children. *Brain and Language*, 1976, *3*, 1-16. (a)

Denckla, M.B., & Rudel, R. Rapid "automatized" naming (R.A.N.): Dyslexia differentiated from other learning disabilities. *Neuropsychologia*, 1976, *14*, 471-479. (b)

deVilliers, J. & deVilliers, P. Delopment of the use of word order in comprehension. *Journal of Psycholinguistic Research*, 1973, *2*, 331-341.

Dixon, N.D. *Reading disability, language impairment and reading strategies: Implications for differential diagnosis*. Unpublished doctoral dissertation, University of Colorado, 1982.

Donohue, M. Learning disabled children's comprehension and production of syntactic devices for making given versus new information. In Chicago Institute for the Study of Learning Disabilities, Abstracts of Research Reports, 1981. (a)

Donohue, M. Requesting strategies of learning disabled children. *Applied Psycholinguistics*, 1981, *2*, 213-234. (b)

Donohue, M., Pearl, R., & Bryan, T. Learning disabled children's conversational competence: Responses to inadequate messages. *Applied Psycholinguistics*, 1980, *1*, 387-404.

Donohue, M., Pearl, R., & Bryan, T. Learning disabled children's syntactic proficiency on a communicative task. *Journal of Speech and Hearing Disorders*, in press.

Dore, J. Conversation and preschool language development. In P. Fletcher & M. Garman (Eds.), *Language acquisition*. Cambridge, Eng.: Cambridge University Press, 1978.

Dunn, L. *Peabody Picture Vocabulary Test*. Circle Pines, MI: American Guidance Services, 1965.

Dunn, L., & Dunn, L. *Peabody Picture Vocabulary Test—Revised*. Circle Pines, MI: American Guidance Services, 1981.

Durrell, J. *The Durrell analysis of reading difficulty*. New York: Harcourt, Brace & Jovanovich, 1965.

Ellis-Weismer, S. *Constructive comprehension processes exhibited by language impaired children*. Unpublished doctoral dissertation, Indiana University, 1981.

Ervin-Tripp, S. Wait for me, roller skate! In S. Ervin-Tripp & C. Mitchell-Kernan (Eds.), *Child discourse*, New York: Academic Press, 1977.

Fillmore, C.J. Types of lexical information. In D.D. Steinberg & L.A. Jakobovits (Eds.), *Semantics: An interdisciplinary reader in philosophy, linguistics and psychology*. Cambridge, Eng: Cambridge University Press, 1971.

Foster, C., Giddan, J., & Stark, J. *Assessment of children's language comprehension*. Palo Alto, CA: Counseling Psychologists Press, 1973.

Freedle, R.O.(Ed.), *Discourse production and comprehension*. Norwood, NJ: Ablex, 1977.

Fry, M.A. *A transformational analysis of the oral language structure used by two reading groups at the second grade level*. Unpublished doctoral dissertation, University of Iowa, 1967.

Fry, M.A., Johnson, C.S., & Muehl, S. Oral language production in relation to reading achievement among select second graders. In D.J. Bakker & P. Satz (Eds.), *Specific reading disability: Advances in theory and method.* Rotterdam: Rotterdam University Press, 1970.

Gallagher, T.M. Revision behaviors in the speech of normal children developing language. *Journal of Speech and Hearing Research,* 1977, *20,* 303-318.

Gardner, R. *One-Word Expressive Vocabulary Test.* Novato, CA: Academic Therapy Publications, 1980.

Garvey, C. Requests andd responses in children's speech. *Journal of Child Language* 1975, *2,* 41-60.

Gelman, R., Bullock, M., & Meck, E. Preschooler's understanding of simple object transformations. *Child Development,* 1980, *51.* 691-699.

German, D.J. Word finding skills in children with learning disabilities. *Journal of Learning Disabilities,* 1979, *12,* 43-48.

Golub, L., & Kidder, C. Syntactic density and the computer, *Elementary English,* 1974, *51,* 1128-1131.

Graybeal, C.M. Memory for stories in language-impaired children. *Applied Psycholinguistics,* 1981, *2,* 269-283.

Greenbaum, S., Quirk, R., Leach, G., & Svartnik, J. *A grammar of contemporary English.* New York: Seminar Press, 1972.

Greenfield, P., & Smith, J. *The structure of communication in early development.* New York: Academic Press, 1976.

Haviland, S.E., & Clark, H.H. What's new? Acquiring new information as a process in comprehension. *Journal of Verbal Learning and Verbal Behavior,* 1974, *13,* 515-521.

Hook, P.E. *A study of metalinguistic awareness and reading strategies in proficient and learning disabled readers.* Unpublished doctoral dissertation, Northwestern University, 1976.

Hornby, P. Surface structure and the topic-comment distinction: A developmental study. *Child Development,* 1971, *42,* 1975-1978.

Hunt, K.W. Grammatical structures written at three grade levels. *National Council of Teachers of English,* No. 3, 1965.

Jansky, J. The marginally reading child. *Bulletin of Orton Society,* 1975, *25,* 69-85.

Johnson, D.J., & Myklebust, H.R. *Learning disabilities: Educational principles and practices.* New York: Grune and Straton, 1967.

Johnson, H., & Smith, L.B. Children's inferential abilities in the context of reading to understand. *Child Development,* 1981, *52,* 1216-1223.

Johnston, J., & Ramstad, V. Cognitive development in preadolescent language-impaired children. Paper presented at the Annual Convention of the American Speech and Hearing Association, Chicago, 1977.

Jorgensen, C., Barrett, M., Huisingh, R., & Zachman, Z. *The Word Test.* Moline, IL.: Lingui Systems, Inc., 1981.

Just, M.N., & Carpenter, P. (Eds.), *Cognitive processes in comprehension.* Hillsdale, NJ: Lawrence Erlbaum Associates, 1977.

Kail, R., Chi, M., Ingram, A., & Danner, F. Constructive aspects of children's reading comprehension. *Child Development,* 1977, *48,* 684-688.

Keenan, J.M., & Kintsch, W. The identification of explicity and implicity presented information. In W. Kintsch, *The representation of meaning in memory.* Hillsdale, NJ: Lawrence Erlbaum Associates, 1974.

Kessel, F.S. The role of syntax in children's comprehension from ages 6 to 12. *Society for Research in Child Development Monograph,* 1970, (Serial No. 139).

Khami, A.G. Nonlinguistic symbolic and conceptual abilities of language-impaired and normally developing children. *Journal of Speech and Hearing Research,* 1981, *24,* 446-453.

Kintsch, E., & Kintsch, W. The comprehension of texts. In R. McLean (Ed.), *Reading.* Belmont, Victoria: Deakin University Press, 1979.

Kintsch, W. *The representation of meaning in memory.* Hillsdale, NJ: Lawrence Erlbaum, 1974.

Kintsch, W. On comprehending stories. In M.A. Just & P. Carpenter (Eds.), *Cognitive processes in comprehension.* Hillsdale, NJ: Lawrence Erlbaum, 1977.

Kintsch, W., & Green, E. The role of culture-specific schemata in the comprehension and recall of stories. *Discourse Processes,* 1979, *1,* 1-13.

Kirk, S., & McCarthy, J. *The Illinois Test of Psycholinguistic Abilities.* Champaign-Urbana: University of Illinois Press, 1961.

Leonard, L.B. What is deviant language? *Journal of Speech and Hearing Disorders,* 1972, *37,* 427-446.

Lerner, J.W. *Children with learning disabilities* Second ed. Boston: Houghton Mifflin, 1977.

Leske, M.C. Speech prevalence estimates of communicative disorders in the U.S. *Asha,* 1981, *23,* 229-237.

Liles, B., Schulman, M., & Bartlett, S. Judgements of grammaticality by normal and language-disordered children. *Journal of Speech and Hearing Disorders,* 1977, *42,* 199-209.

Mandler, J.M., & Johnson, N.S. Remembrance of things parsed: Story structure and recall. *Cognitive Psychology,* 1977, *9,* 111-151.

Mattis, S., French, J., & Rapin, I. Dyslexia in children and young adults: Three independent neurological syndromes. *Developmental Medicine and Child Neurology,* 1975, *17,* 150-163.

Moran, M.R., & Byrne, M.C. Mastery of verb tense markers by normal and learning disabled children. *Journal of Speech and Hearing Research,* 1977, *20,* 529-542.

Meline, T. Referential communication by normal and language deficient children. Paper presented at the annual convention of the American Speech and Hearing Association, San Francisco, 1978.

Murphy, V.H. *A comparison of four measures of visual imagery in normal and language disorderd children.* Unpublished master's thesis, Northern Illinois University, 1978.

Murphy, V.H., & Stephens, M.I. A comparison of four measures of visual imagery in normal and language disordered children. In preparation.

Newcomer, P., & Hammill, D. *Test of Language Development.* Austin, TX: Empiric Press, 1977.

Paris, S., & Upton, L. Children's memory for inferential relationships in prose. *Child Development,* 1976, *47,* 660-668.

Piaget, J., & Inhelder, B. *Mental imagery in the child.* New York: Basic Books, 1971.

Prinz, P. The comprehension and production of requests in language disordered children. Paper presented at the Second Annual Boston University Conference on Language Development, Boston, October 1977.

Prinz, P. Requesting in normal and language disordered children. In K. Nelson (Ed.), *Children's language* (Vol. 3). New York: Gardner Press, in press.

Riley, C., & Trabasso, T. Comparatives, logical structures, and encoding in a transitive inference task. *Journal of Experimental Child Psychology,* 1974, *17,* 187-203.

Rumelhardt, D.E. Schemata: The building blocks of cognition. In R.J. Spiro, B.C. Bruce, & W.F. Brewer (Eds.), *Theoretical issues in reading comprehension.* Hillsdale, NJ: Lawrence Erlbaum, 1980.

Savich, P.A. *A comparison of the anticipatory imagery and spatial representation ability of normal and language disordered children.* Unpublished doctoral dissertation, University of Colorado, 1980.

Schulte, C. *A study of the relationship between oral language and reading achiement in second graders.* Unpublished doctoral dissertation, University of Iowa, 1967.

Schank, R.C., & Abelson, R.P. *Scripts, plans, goals and understanding.* Hillsdale, NJ: Lawrence Erlbaum, 1977.

Semel, E., & Wiig, E. Comprehension of syntactic structures and critical verbal elements by children with learning disabilities. *Journal of Learning Disabilities,* 1975, *8,* 53-58.

Shatz, M. On the development of communicative understanding: An early strategy for interpreting and responding to messages. *Cognitive Psychology,* 1978, *10,* 217-301.

Sheppard, L. Evolution of the identification of perceptual-cognitive disorders in Colorado. Final Report. Boulder: Laboratory of Educational Research, University of Colorado, 1981.

Snyder, L.S., Haas, C., & Becker, L.B. Discourse processing in normal and language and learning disabled children. Unpublished manuscript, 1982.

Stark, R., & Tallal, P. Selection of children with specific language deficits. *Journal of Speech and Hearing Disorders,* 1981, *46,* 114-122.

Stein, N., & Glenn, C. An analysis of story comprehension in elementary school children. In R. Freedle (Ed.), *New directions in discourse processing.* Hillsdale, NJ: Ablex, 1979.

Strauss, A., & Lehtinen, L. *Psychopathology and education of the brain-injured child.* New York: Grune & Stratton, 1946.

Trabasso, T. Representation, memory and reasoning: How do we make transitive inferences? In A. Pick (Ed.), *Minnesota Symposium on Child Psychology* (Vol. 9). Minneapolis: University of Minnesota Press, 1975.

Trabasso, T., & Nicholas, D. Memory and inferences in the comprehension of narratives. Paper presented at the Conference on Study of Children's Judgements, Kassel, Germany, June 1977.

U.S. Office of Education. Assistance to states for handicapped children. Procedure for evaluating specific learning disabilities. *Federal Register,* 1977, *42,* 65082-65085.

Vogel, S.A. *Syntactic abilities in normal and dyslexic children.* Baltimore: University Park Press, 1975.

Vogel, S. Syntactic abilities in normal and dyslexic children. *Journal of Learning Disabilities,* 1977, *7,* 47-53.

Weaver, P., & Dickenson, D. Story comprehension and recall in dyslexic students. *Bulletin of Orton Society,* 1979, *29,* 157-171.

Wiig, E.H., & Semel, E.M. Comprehension of linguistic concepts requiring logical operations by learning disabled children. *Journal of Speech and Hearing Research,* 1973, *16,* 627-636.

Wiig, E.H., & Semel, E.M. *Language disabilities in children and adolescents.* Columbus, OH: Charles C. Merrill, 1976.

Wiig, E.H., & Semel, E.M. *Language assessment and intervention for the learning disabled.* Columbus, OH.: Charles E. Merrill, 1980.

Wiig, E.H., & Semel, E.M. *Clinical evaluation of language function.* Columbus, OH.: Charles E. Merrill, 1981.

Wiig, E.H., Semel, E.M., & Crouse, M.B. The use of English morphology by high-risk and learning disabled children. *Journal of Learning Disabilities,* 1973, *6,* 457-465.

Wiig, E.H., Semel, E.M., & Nystrom, L.A. Comparison of rapid naming abilities in language learning disabled and academically achieving eight-year-olds. *Language, Speech and Hearing Services in the Schools,* 1982, *13,* 11-23.

Wolf, M. The relationship of word-finding and reading in children and aphasics. Unpublished doctoral dissertation, Harvard University, 1979.

Elizabeth M. Prather

Developmental Language Disorders: Adolescents

When asked to write this chapter on adolescent language disorders, I could think only of the many unknowns. For the past five years, I have gathered considerable information on the language of the adolescent, including normative data, differential diagnoses, and clinical treatment. Yet, we clinicians still seem like "babes in the woods," perhaps similar to our state 20 years ago regarding childhood language development and disorders. I have accepted the challenge of writing this chapter, not so much from the standpoint of what we know but from that of what we don't know, and in the belief that it may stimulate much needed research.

Normative Data—A Description of Language in Older Children and Adolescents

The discussion in this chapter is limited to students from fifth and sixth grades to the twelfth grade. The normative data have all been derived from standardized tests, and some are much more complete than others. We will see that from ages 11 to 18 years, some characteristics of language commonly show no improvement or change in development. Others demonstrate marked change, while yet others have not been investigated at the adolescent level.

© College-Hill Press, Inc. All rights, including that of translation, reserved. No part of this publication may be reproduced without the written permission of the publisher.

Language Similarities from
Upper Elementary to High School

There is little evidence to suggest that students in high school perform appreciably better on language tests (from the view of speech-language pathology) than students in fifth and sixth grades. Two explanations probably account for this lack of change in test scores. First, current tests may be insensitive to the progress students make in language facility from fifth grade to high school. In other words, we may be testing the wrong factors. Second, there is the possibility that little changes in the student's ability to manipulate some aspects of language meaningfully beyond at least the fifth grade level. This latter possibility may reflect either a plateau or the upper end of certain language rule learning. We would, of course, expect increases in vocabulary as a result of content teaching in classroom curricula, and in the social use of language because of the growing importance of the peer group, but, perhaps, skills like repeating sentences verbatim, understanding subtle syntactic changes, and explaining the meaning of a known concept do not substantially increase during adolescence.

A review of current clinical language tests, all published in 1980, indicates little progress in students' abilities from the upper elementary to the high-school level, as exemplified in the following two screening tests and two more complete diagnostic batteries.

On the *Clinical Evaluation of Language Function Advanced Level Screening Test* (Semel & Wiig, 1980b), the mean number of items passed by fifth-grade students was 35.2, while the mean number passed by twelfth-grade students was only 39.6 from a total of 52 items. Tenth-grade students earned a mean score of only 35.1, slightly lower than fifth-grade. This total increase of approximately four items in seven years should be considered minimal.

Prather, Breecher, Stafford, and Wallace (1980) showed, on the *Screening Test of Adolescent Language* (STAL), that fifth-grade students earned a mean of 14.81 items, while ninth-grade students earned a mean score of 17.86. Most of the improvement resulted from the vocabulary subtest. The increase of essentially 3 items (from a total of 23 items) spans a four-year period, and indicates only slightly better sensitivity to change.

Semel and Wiig (1980b) devised their screening test from a more comprehensive diagnostic battery, *Clinical Evaluation of Language Function* (CELF) (1980a). As of this writing, the CELF does not include means and standard deviations for each grade level, but does show a "criterion score" for each grade level on each of the 13 subtests. The criterion scores are used to determine whether further "extension testing" is needed, reflecting perhaps a lower limit of normal performance for students at each grade level. On 6 of the 13 subtests, *no change* is reflected in the criterion scores from the sixth through the twelfth grades. On the other 7 subtests, the change varies from 2 items (2 subtests) to 4 items (2 subtests) to 8 items (3 subtests). The 3 subtests reflecting the greatest change, approximately one point per year, are as follows:

1. Processing relationships and ambiguities. Examples resemble:
    a. Mary followed Joe, and Joe followed Ann.
       Did Ann follow Mary?
    b. Better late than never. Does it mean: Don't
       be late?
2. Producing word associations. This task requires the student to name as many words as possible within two categories, and is timed.
3. Producing model sentences. The student repeats both meaningful and nonmeaningful "sentences" verbatim.

"Producing formulated sentences" is one of the subtests on which there is no change from sixth through twelfth grades. In this subtest, the student is given 12 words and asked to make a meaningful sentence with each. She or he can receive up to 8 points per sentence, depending on grammatic/syntactic complexity. A score of 3 is given to a simple sentence with phrase(s). The criterion score for this subtest is 35 for all seven grade levels, just under an average of 3 points per sentence. This lack of change over the 7 years is interesting in light of the ways speech-language pathologists program language-delayed students to use complex, compound, and embedded sentences. Perhaps if we knew more about "normal language" in adolescents, we would alter many of our current treatment goals.

The *Test of Adolescent Language* (TOAL) (Hammill, Brown, Larsen, & Wiederholt, 1980) includes normative data from ages 11 to 18½ years, also a span of 7 years. This more complete diagnostic test includes eight subtests of vocabulary and grammar across the four dimensions of listening, speaking, reading, and writing. It is not surprising that students show relatively less growth on the 4 grammar subtests than on the 4 vocabulary subtests, reaffirming the premise that syntactic/grammatic skills are well established by the eleventh birthday in normally developing students. The total change in group means between 11 and 18½ years in the speaking/grammar subtest (repeating sentences verbatim) was 2.3 more items correct in the 7-year span. Among the four dimensions, listening and speaking scores increased less than reading and, especially, writing scores. This result would also be expected if one assumes that the hierarchy of language development proceeds from listening to speaking to reading to writing. The normal developmental period for the reading and writing dimensions of language seems to extend at least into the teen years.

In summary, the clinical tests we are using lack sensitivity to change in the reception and expression of oral language from ages 11 to 18 years. We apparently cannot use existing tests to detect changes in many of the syntactic, grammatic, and memory aspects of language that are tested so heavily at earlier age levels.

Language Differences from Upper Elementary to High School

Evidence is available from other standardized tests that language facility indeed increases among students from fifth through twelfth grades. One very obvious example is that of vocabulary. On the *Peabody Picture Vocabulary Test—Revised Form L* (Dunn & Dunn, 1981), a raw score of 114 converts to an age-equivalent score of 11 years. In contrast, a raw score of 150 converts to an age-equivalent score of 18 years, 1 month. In other words, the high-school senior is expected to identify approximately 36 more items than the fifth-grader, a substantial increase. The more difficult items include terms from the study of geography, mathematics, anatomy, and physics, as well as less common adjectives and verbs.

Performance on the verbal scale of the *Wechsler Intelligence Scale for Children* (WISC) (1949) also shows considerable change from age 11 years to the ceiling age (15 years, 11 months) on 4 of the 6 subtests. The greatest increase is on the vocabulary subtest, which requires the student to define words orally. Many of the high-level, less common words would be known through academic coursework, readings, or exposure to specific experiences, i.e., *hara-kiri, ballast, mantis,* and *chattel.* The information subtest also increases in expectation from ages 11 to 16. The increase reflects greater knowledge, primarily in the areas of geography, history, and the sciences.

Two additional subtests of the WISC, general comprehension and similarities, show some change, but less than vocabulary and information. The general comprehension subtest, except for the 4 lowest-level items, requires the student to answer "why" questions (cause-effect relationships) of increasing difficulty. The similarities subtest (identifying key components of likeness) increases in difficulty for the older student by the inclusion of more abstract concepts, for example, *liberty-justice, first-last,* and *49-121.*

The two subtests of the WISC which show essentially no increase across the five years are arithmetic and digit span. The arithmetic items, beyond the low-level, block manipulations, are all short "story problems," which the subject hears (10 items) or reads (3 items). All require only basic arithmetic concepts of addition, subtraction, multiplication, and division of whole numbers or fractions. The digit-span task for auditory memory is scored by adding the number of digits correctly recalled on the two tasks of forward and backward repetition. The average 11-year-old student earns a score of ten digits (perhaps six forward and four backward) while the 15- to 16-year-old student earns a score of eleven digits. This failure to see an increase in memory span resembles the sentence-repetition performances described earlier in other language tests.

Other evidence in language growth through the teen years can be found in the various school achievement tests used throughout the country (*Peabody Individualized Achievement Test,* Dunn & Markwardt, 1970; *California Achievement Tests,* CTB/McGraw-Hill, 1977; *Wide Range Achievement Test,* Jastak, 1946; and *Metropolitan Achievement Tests,* Prescott, Balow, Hogan, & Farr, 1978). All of these tests measure various aspects of reading and vocabulary, and are dependent on academic achievement.

In summary, tests of vocabulary, abstract-concept explanations, and general knowledge of academic content areas show marked improvement in scores from the fifth to the twelfth grades, and reflect the expected semantic growth resulting from increased reading and exposure to many learning experiences. Curricular materials from classrooms at various grade levels reflect this semantic development.

Language Processes Not Yet Described

To my knowledge, no standardized tests for adolescents are available that tap pragmatic aspects of language, including topic maintenance, sensitivity to misunderstandings, and group problem-solving strategies. We certainly can predict that changes are expected in these areas as well as other areas related to the social use of language as the peer group gains importance. Much research is needed to identify and quantify some of the key components of language usage among adolescents.

Assessing Expected Competencies Among Adolescents

Clinicians would like to find discreet types of language disorders among adolescents. In theory, such findings would simplify remedial programming. Just as there are many dimensions of language, we can assume that there are also many possible dimensions to language disorders evidenced singly and in combination. We can also assume that there are as many etiological variables affecting language performance in adolescents as there are in younger children and adults.

No one questions the evidence that students who are mentally retarded, severely and multiply handicapped, autistic, hearing-impaired, and/or brain-damaged from trauma are likely to have difficulty manipulating the code system of language. We do, however, assume that the specific configuration of difficulties will differ both within and across etiological categories. Likewise, to expect that we can find a few distinct "types" of language problems in adolescents has to be totally unrealistic.

A group of special interest is the "learning disabled." I call it a "group" because, by educational placement, these students are apparently assumed to share at least some common characteristics. McGrady (1980, pp. 509-562) presents an excellent discussion on the diverse ways in which the term "learning disability" has been used and defined. He points out that, through use of behavioral testing, we now see school districts claiming 5% to 20% or more of their students as learning disabled. This incidence is in sharp contrast to the 1 to 2 % of students expected to have neurologically significant specific learning disabilities. The difference, according to McGrady, is that many students who are simply "underachievers and slow learners" have been labeled as "learning disabled." Many of these students are merely victims of poor teaching, or have come from families that do not value academic achievement. To expect that large segments of these students will have a specific "type" of language disability (e.g., poor auditory memory, language-processing problems, auditory figure-ground confusions, morphological/syntactical problems, word retrieval problems) is unrealistic, even if we could isolate and define the parameters of such specific deficits.

Assessment among adolescents includes at least two discrete tasks. The first is screening to determine which students need a more complete diagnostic evaluation. The second is the evaluation used to (1) determine whether a communication problem exists; (2) document the language disorder; and (3) program remedial or compensatory training.

Language Screening

Screening students for all types of communication disorders is an important task in school settings. In some districts, routine screening occurs at certain grade levels, while in other districts more reliance is placed on teacher and parent referrals.

Screening protocols for language among older students have posed real problems for us. Because of the lack of normative data, clinicians have relied heavily on short "informal" dialogues and monologues. Asking students such questions as "How many brothers and sisters do you have? What are their names and ages? How long have you lived in Phoenix?" is useless if used with this older age group to identify possible language problems. These questions are typically answered well by students in the primary grades. Simple monologues also may be equally ineffective. In an early draft of the STAL (Prather et al., 1980), we had included a subtest that required the student to relate a story from sequenced picture cues. We had to eliminate the subtest because of our inability to attain scoring reliability among various examiners. Some examiners gave maximum credit to a story told with correct grammar, paying little attention to content elaboration, complexity of sentence structure, or the sequencing of ideas. Some of these informal approaches for language screening, then, are no doubt ineffective, and result in highly variable judgments within and between school districts. To my knowledge, no researchers have extended the work of O'Donnell, Griffin, and Norris (1967) on T-Unit norms from the elementary to the high-school level, nor have the six production indices used by Ludlow (1977, pp. 97-134) with adult asphasics been normed on adolescents. Such approaches might be worthwhile.

One mini-screening test (Prather, Brenner, & Hughes, 1981), requiring approximately 90 seconds per student, has been devised for the mass screening of older students. It includes five items: two in vocabulary, one in sentence repetition, one in explanation of cause-effect, and one in sentence explanation. The normative data indicate that the test passes approximately 75% of students from regular classrooms (sixth to twelfth grades). Additional screening time can then be spent with the 25% who fail.

Two more complete language-screening tests are available for use with adolescents. Both provide a standardized protocol for screening, and both tap several aspects of language. The STAL (Prather et al., 1980) requires approximately 7 minutes per student, while the Advanced Level CELF Screening Test (Semel & Wiig, 1980b) requires approximately 15 minutes. A student may "fail" either screening test because of poor performance on any one subtest, or because of a low total score. Both tests seem useful in identifying students whose language skills differ markedly from their peers and who may profit from more complete assessment.

Speech-Language Evaluations

Two excellent sources on expected language competencies are available (Bassett, Wittington, & Staton-Spicer, 1978; Simon, 1979). Both force the clinician to focus on specific features of speaking and listening that require assessment. Bassett et al. suggest guidelines for minimal speaking and listening competencies for high-school graduates, and urge that we assess not memorized facts, but the students' ability to use speaking and listening skills for tasks encountered in adult living. They divide 19 competencies among four areas. The first area is the use of the verbal and nonverbal codes to understand and express meaning. It includes such skills as understanding directions, using language appropriate to given situations, speaking clearly and loudly enough to be heard and understood, and using nonverbal signs (gestures and facial expressions) that are appropriate to the situation. The second assesses understanding of oral messages and includes skills such as identification of the main idea in messages; distinguishing fact from opinion, and information from persuasion; and recognizing when another has not understood your message. The third area measures elements selected and arranged to produce spoken messages. It includes skills such as expressing ideas clearly and concisely, defending a point of view, sequencing information so that others can understand, asking questions to obtain information, giving accurate and concise directions, and summarizing messages. Their last area looks at resolving conflicts in human relationships, and includes skills that can be assessed as describing another's point of view and differences of opinion, expressing feelings to others, and performing social rituals.

To assess all of these functional communication skills suggested by Bassett et al. (1978) requires that we approach assessment from a pragmatic level. They do not, however, include any suggestions for formal assessment. Simon (1979) not only presents a model for expressive communicative competence, but also suggests ways to obtain evidence of competence and incompetence. The reader is strongly urged to refer directly to Simon's Appendix 4, pages 69-76. It is filled with suggested activities for observing a student's use of language, including the seven functions of language as described by Halliday. These are: instrumental, regulatory, interactional, personal, heuristic, imaginative, and informational. In addition, Simon's battery includes phonology, morphology, syntax, semantics, and a few suggestions for observing receptive language. Her suggested approaches to the evaluation and treatment of language problems are not limited to the adolescent level; she includes much information on younger children as well. She has, however, incorporated many suggestions specific to the intermediate and junior high-school level.

In addition to specifying which aspects of language need to be tested, and how each might be observed, Simon (1979) also provides a system to organize accumulated data on each student, so that the strengths and weaknesses in speech and language become evident. She uses some standardized test scores to include with the documentation of the need for speech-language services. She agrees, however, with Leonard, Prutting, Perozzi and Berkley (1978), who advocate use of informal, descriptive evaluation procedures for communicative competence, and she states that our knowledge of the nature of effective communication exceeds our development of formal evaluation instruments. Thus, her format for organizing assessment information and writing comprehensive treatment objectives is a strong contribution to the working clinician.

Two recent diagnostic measures previously mentioned in this chapter— CELF and TOAL— are now available for use with adolescents. However, neither provides the types of functional assessment advocated by Simon (1979) and Bassett et al. (1978). Both the CELF and the TOAL are designed to reflect various patterns of strengths and weaknesses. The CELF includes 13 subtests across many aspects of receptive and expressive language. Normative data are severely limited in this first edition, and the test protocol does not provide for basal and ceiling scores. With some students, the need to administer all items in each subtest seems unnecessarily redundant.

The TOAL does provide basal and ceiling scores for its 8 subtests; administration time, however, ranges from one to three hours per student. The test is especially helpful to those clinicians who want language measures related to reading and writing (4 of the 8 subtests). Many of the listening and speaking test items are constructed to reduce guessing by requiring the two most appropriate choices from a set of four or five foils.

No assessment tools of interactive communication have been standardized on adolescents at this time. We can hope that research is under way which will help the clinician identify and assess those competencies that are expected in adolescent students. It may be possible to start a standardized functional communication procedure for adolescents with the *Communication Abilities in Daily Living* (Holland, 1980), capitalizing on her previous research with adult aphasics.

In addition to the observations and tests used to assess language competence, other school personnel and records are helpful. Besides the classroom teacher, the psychologist and counselor are especially important. Psychometric data and achievement test scores may be particularly helpful in understanding the nature of a possible language problem.

Treatment with Older Language-Impaired Students

Can language problems be remediated at these older age levels, or should we attempt to teach compensatory and coping strategies? In a possibly parallel situation, Darley (1972) wrote a treatise on the efficacy of language rehabilitation with aphasic adults. He concluded at that time that no generalizations to the population of aphasic patients was possible, and urged that future investigations specify the nature of the language problem treated, the objective measurement of relevant behavioral changes, and the nature, intensity, and quality of therapy provided. Darley's article, though over 10 years old, and directed to the effectiveness of treatment with aphasic patients, is applicable today to the treatment of language disorders in adolescents. Essentially no data for the latter population, beyond case studies, are available, however. The nature of the language problems has not been identified, the measurements for change have been gross, and the definitions of treatment inadequate.

The nature of treatment varies greatly across our field. The need for an individualized educational plan for each student suggests that it varies depending on the needs, strengths, and weaknesses of each individual. Yet, variability in approaches far exceeds student differences. It is not possible to include a thorough discussion of treatment in the context of this chapter, but a few of the major issues should be mentioned.

1. **Teaching to the student's weakness vs teaching to the student's strengths.** Teaching to the weaknesses suggests that (a) it is possible to determine the underlying nature of the language problem through diagnostic tests, and (b) remediation techniques are, or can be, effective in eliminating or greatly reducing the underlying problem. One is reminded here of programs designed to increase auditory memory or auditory processing based on the hypothesis that weaknesses in these areas have caused the problem. Two sources (Hammill & Larsen, 1974; Rees, 1981) are especially enlightening on the limited payoff of such approaches.

Teaching to the strengths suggests that (a) it is possible to determine the aspects of language the student handles well; and (b) remediation techniques that capitalize on these strengths will help the student compensate for the weaknesses. Such approaches always start with what the student "can do" and build to higher levels of achievement through progressive *successes*.

2. **Listening and speaking vs listening, speaking, reading, and writing.** The role of the clinician in treatment of reading and writing disorders is not clear. Whether we believe we should, or should not, be involved in the teaching of reading and written language depends heavily on personal philosophies, education, and experiences. For the most part, however, our training institutions are failing to ensure background in the areas of reading and written language.

3. **Syntactic-grammatic emphasis vs conceptual-semantic emphasis.** The ease with which syntax and grammar can be tested and programmed, and the changes documented, has probably resulted in a heavy grammatic emphasis in treatment programs. We know far less about which

concepts precede others in normal development (especially at the older age levels), or how to teach "concepts."

4. Language "brain twisters" vs functional communication. Many language "exercises" have been developed, even though the student rarely has an opportunity to use the new skill. I am reminded of a mother who recently brought her 14-year-old daughter to our clinic for service. This mother desired functional language skills, like answering the phone and taking accurate messages, rather than the learning of what "raining cats and dogs" means, an unusable skill, in her opinion, which the previous clinician had emphasized.

5. Motivation problems. It is a common complaint among clinicians that older students neither want their services nor are motivated for improvement. Furthermore, some say that services at the high-school level are not crucial, because students, once scheduled, do not show up for treatment sessions. All of us have failed at times to relate to and motivate the older student, usually one who has had several years of previous experience in speech-language therapy.

It seems obvious that students who are discouraged because of lack of progress would like to stop what has become a defeating and punishing experience. I have heard students state openly that "Speech therapy has not helped before, why would it help now?" Some have been forced to drill in areas of weakness, which has amplified their feelings of failure. We recently worked with a young college student who had many years of treatment, along with placement in a self-contained learning-disability classroom. For the past six years, he had struggled unsuccessfully to increase his auditory and visual memory span. At the time he entered our clinic, he presented a severe communication problem, including: lack of eye contact even on an occasional basis; a slow monotonous rate of speech, with frequent sentence revisions and interjections; very poor intelligibility, resulting from reduced mouth opening and limited articulatory movements; and no seeming desire to attempt changes. Any confidence he once had as a speaker had apparently been obliterated by inappropriate prior treatment, and the severity of his communication problem had increased rather than decreased.

Most students who truly have a communication disorder *and* hold the belief that speech-language therapy will be beneficial do not have motivation or attendance problems. An approach that I have used with considerable success might be termed the "three-week bargain." It involves a student-clinician agreement to commit themselves to three weeks of effort prior to rejecting the service. The clinician then must target and program for a high level of success on a change that is important to the student, not one that seemingly has no application to his or her life. Students often will discuss changes that *they* would like to make and the clinician might wisely heed their words.

Not all clinicians relate well with older students, just as some fail with preschoolers, and others with adults. Those who work well with adolescents seem to relate in straightforward, honest ways, avoiding false enthusiasm and condensension. Students are treated like adults and the responsibility for change is placed directly with them, not the parents.

It is not possible at this time to document the effectiveness of any of the above treatment approaches from controlled research. Logic, however, suggests that some approaches make more sense than others. If treatment is effective, then those approaches that help an individual student communicate in daily life seem preferable. If treatment is ineffective, why work to perfect skills in verbal exercises like repeating word strings, rearranging words from cut-up written sentences, or defining obscure and rarely used idioms?

Logic also suggests that we capitalize on each student's strengths and use those strengths to compensate as much as possible for weaknesses. For example, students can be encouraged to use short simple sentences effectively, rather than be forced to produce complex and embedded sentences which, for them, are meaningless.

Some clinicians organize the content of their treatment programs almost entirely from classroom curricula. From a logical standpoint, this simple approach seems excellent. It is very easy for them to obtain desk copies of the texts used at various grade levels. Many topics are covered at several intervals throughout the curriculum; for example, state history may be introduced in the fourth grade, and continued in the seventh and tenth grades. Using materials from the lower grade levels may be appropriate with students who do not have the basic concepts on which the new material is based. Content for all language targets (vocabulary, grammar, discourse, verbal explanations, cause-effect relationships, etc.) can be taken from the topics currently being studied in the student's classroom. From my discussions with many school clinicians, it almost seems as if this basic approach to treatment is so obvious that it is often overlooked. We state that language problems interfere with academic success. If so, then it seems advisable to program treatment using content on which academic success will be measured. The lack of normative data on expected competencies also supports use of school curricular materials. Moreover, such materials contain the vocabulary and concepts expected at the various grade levels.

Finally, the issue of teaching various subskills versus teaching directly to the problem needs comment. Perhaps you have heard about the reading teacher who started remediation with the sixth-grader by doing arm muscle exercises to increase his ability to hold a book. I hope we are less ridiculous.

Until we have evidence to the contrary, the shortest, most direct approach to a functional target is preferred.

Summary

From the foregoing discussion, we have seen that research data on adolescent language disorders are limited. Standardized test results from speech-language pathology, psychology, and education were used to describe language skills in older students and adolescents. In the areas of syntax, grammar, and auditory memory, test results indicate little improvement among normally developing students beyond the fifth-grade level. The semantic aspects of language, on the other hand, increase markedly between the fifth and twelfth grades. This increase in vocabulary, abstract concept development, and general knowledge is expected from academic curricula, extended reading, and exposure to many learning experiences. In other areas of language, specifically pragmatics and the social use of language, no normative research data are available to document expected competencies across the adolescent years.

The assessment and treatment of expected competencies with the older, language-impaired student were also discussed. The lack of research greatly hinders our ability to recommend specific procedures or protocols. I have attempted, however, to suggest that we emphasize *functional* communication skills both in assessment and treatment. Such an approach says that if our intervention makes a difference, it will be in those aspects of language the student encounters in daily living. By using content material from classroom curricula, for example, students are exposed to the vocabulary and concepts needed for school achievement—those with which they are likely to be more familiar.

References

Bassett, R.E., Whittington, N. & Staton-Spicer, A. The basics in speaking and listening for high-school graduates: What should be assessed? *Communication Education,* 1978, *27,* 293-303.

The California Achievement Tests. Monterey, CA: CTB/McGraw-Hill, 1977.

Darley, F.L. The efficacy of language rehabilitation in aphasia. *Journal of Speech and Hearing Disorders,* 1972, *37,* 3-21.

Dunn, Lloyd M., & Dunn, Leota M. *Peabody Picture Vocabulary Test—Revised* (Form L). Circle Pines, MN: American Guidance Service, 1981.

Dunn, L.M., & Markwardt, F.C. *Peabody Individualized Achievement Test.* Circle Pines, MN: American Guidance Service, 1970.

172   Prather

Hammill, D.D., Brown, V.L., Larsen, S.C., & Wiederholt, J.L. *Test of Adolescent Language: A Multidimensional Approach to Assessment.* Austin, TX: Services for Professional Educators, 1980.

Hammill, D.D., & Larsen, S.C. The effectiveness of psycholinguistic training. *Exceptional Children,* 1974, *40,* 5-14.

Holland, A. *Communicative abilities in daily living.* Baltimore: University Park Press, 1980.

Jastak, J. *Wide Range Achievement Test.* Wilmington, DE: Charles L. Story, 1946.

Leonard, L.B., Prutting, C., Perozzi, J.A., & Berkley, R.K. Nonstandardized approaches to the assessment of language behaviors. *Asha,* 1978, *20,* 371-397.

Ludlow, C. Recovery from aphasia: A foundation for treatment. In M. Sullivan & M.S. Kommers (Eds.), *Rationale for adult aphasia therapy.* Omaha: University of Nebraska Medical Center, 1977.

McGrady, H.J. Communication disorders in specific learning disabilities. In R.J. Van Hattam (Ed.), *Communication disorders: An introduction.* New York: Macmillan, 1980.

O'Donnell, P.D., Griffin, W.J., & Norris, R.C. Syntax of kindergarten and elementary school children: A transformational analysis. Research Report No. 8. NCTE Committee on Research, 508 S. 6th Street, Champaign, IL, 1967.

Prather, E.M., Breecher, S.V., Stafford, M.L., & Wallace, E.M. *Screening Test of Adolescent Language* (STAL). Seattle: University of Washington Press, 1980.

Prather, E.M., Brenner, A.C., & Hughes, K.S. A mini-screening language test for adolescents. *Language, Speech, and Hearing Services in Schools,* 1981, *12,* 67-73.

Prescott, G.A., Balow, I.H., Hogan, T.P., & Farr, R.C. *Metropolitan Achievement Tests: Survey Battery.* New York: Psychological Corp., 1978.

Rees, N. Saying more than we know: Is auditory processing disorder a meaningful concept? In R. Keith, *Central auditory and language disorders in children.* San Diego: College-Hill Press, 1981.

Semel, E., & Wiig, E. *Clinical Evaluation of Language Function* (CELF). Columbus, OH: Charles E. Merrill, 1980. (a)

Semel, E., & Wiig, E. *Clinial Evaluation of Language Function Advanced Level Screening Test.* Columbus, OH: Charles E. Merrill, 1980. (b)

Simon, C.S. *Communicative competence: A functional-pragmatic approach to language therapy.* Tucson, AZ: Communication Skills Builders, 1979.

Wechsler, D. *Wechsler Intelligence Scale for Children* (WISC). New York: Psychological Corporation, 1949.

Marie Capozzi
Beth Mineo

Nonspeech Language and Communication Systems

The emergence of nonspeech communication as a unique discipline is a recent phenomenon. Although estimates concerning the birth of this discipline vary, it is safe to say that most of the influential developments have occurred in the last decade. The complex and varied needs of the nonspeaking population—those who cannot manage a productive system of spoken language (Schiefelbusch & Hollis, 1980) —require that speech and language clinicians be "renaissance people," knowledgeable not only in all aspects of speech and language development, but also in psychology, child development, physical therapy, occupational therapy, and, to some degree, in engineering, computer science, and design.

This relatively new discipline, once regarded as peddling "gadgetry," is finally gaining the respect and recognition it deserves. The goal of the nonspeech-language interventionist is to facilitate independent communication for nonspeakers of all ages, physical abilities, and cognitive levels. This does not mean that every person will be handed a microprocessor-based system and be expected to say something movingly profound. It does mean that we have at our disposal a wide range of devices—some extremely simple and others employing quite sophisticated technology— and a wealth of information gained from recent research which allows us to provide services that have a lasting impact on our clients.

Professional organizations and a limited number of universities have begun to acknowledge the discipline and its accomplishments. We stress

© College-Hill Press, Inc. All rights, including that of translation, reserved. No part of this publication may be reproduced without the written permission of the publisher.

the importance of this chapter's information for all speech and language clinicians—for nonspeakers are found in schools, hospitals, and private clinics. In many instances, the clinician must not only fulfill the typical role, but is often required to serve as the co-ordinator of a transdisciplinary habilitation/rehabilitation team. Although this chapter has application for clinicians working with the entire range of communicatively handicapped persons, its primary focus is the assessment of and subsequent intervention with school-aged children who have not acquired vocal speech due to cognitive delay, and those who cannot functionally communicate via the vocal channel due to neuromuscular involvement, i.e., cerebral palsy, head trauma, or degenerative disease.

We tend to take speech for granted until we are forced to deal with its absence, as in the case of aphasia or debilitating and/or progressive dysarthria. Consider, on the other hand, the child born with so severe a physical disability that he or she is not only precluded from developing speech, but also from motorically manipulating the world. From infancy, the establishment of bonding relationships through feeding, sucking, and vocalizing are disrupted. The physical impairment interferes with the child's ability to "make something happen in his world" (Morris, 1981) by exploration and manipulation of toys and objects through mouthing, kicking, pushing, hitting, etc. Further, severely handicapped children have difficulty evoking vocal and physical feedback from parents and others. Parent interactions which are

> normally warm and rewarding may become situations of frustration and tension for caregivers who are uncomfortable in dealing with the physically handicapped child's erratic, involuntary, and spastic or athetoid reflexive movements. Motor-related handicaps can thus result in social/emotional, interactional, motivational, and communicative handicaps (Harris-Vanderheiden, 1976, p. 235).

As a result of this "experiental deprivation" (Goodenough-Trepagnier & Prather, 1981, p. 323), it is our belief that the conceptual formulations of these children differ from those of normal children, although comprehensive and early intervention to facilitate prelinguistic and linguistic achievement may alter these differences.

Many factors contribute to the decision to augment a child's communication. Primary among these is the inability to speak; other factors, such as physical and cognitive abilities, are vital in determining the type of augmentative system to be prescribed. Decisions about candidate selection and the intervention techniques used in designing and developing a communication system are generally contingent on analyzing the child's linguistic, cognitive, and physical status. Abilities in these areas cover a wide range, and each child presents unique combinations of strengths and weaknesses. For example, at Pioneer Center (a Pittsburgh public school for multiply handicapped children), there is Jennifer, a bright and very social 13-year-old, who has severe cerebral palsy along with cognitive and educational levels that are generally age-appropriate. Diana, another cerebral-palsied nonspeaker, is not only severely motorically and visually impaired, but also is cognitively handicapped. In contrast to these two severely physically handicapped students, Janice has full control over her hands and oral structures, yet fails to be an effective functional communicator due to profound mental retardation.

The purpose of this chapter is to: (1) describe the assessment procedures vital for determining a nonspeaking child's present level of functioning in both physical and communication realms, (2) review methods of intervention towards the goal of independent communication, and (3) acquaint the reader with trends in the development of communication devices.

Assessment Aspects

Physical Status

The physical assessment evaluates the child's ability to control and coordinate movement patterns. The precision with which these patterns are executed is inversely related to severity of impairment. Children who display minimal motor dysfunction have increased options in selecting and using efficient communication systems. Examples include children whose oral structures may be moderately involved, and whose oral speaking can be characterized as functional in a variety of settings. Other children may not be functional oral speakers, but can maintain efficient-to-adequate control of the upper extremities (hands, fingers), allowing for the development of "signing" systems. The children addressed in this section have physical conditions that result in severe motoric disabilities of the oral channel, thereby precluding the development of independent functional speech. These severely handicapped children are unable to inhibit abnormal reflexes and involuntary muscle action, and to coordinate and control muscle movement patterns necessary for normal communication acquisition.

A transdisciplinary team usually is responsible for assessing the motor functioning of physically handicapped children. Speech pathologists, along with physical and occupational therapists, assess the physical status of the child, and determine muscle function capabilities for using communication and environmental control devices. In addition, physical and occupational therapists are responsible for the child's correct positioning in different situations, i.e., in standing tables, on a prone board, on a mat, in a travel chair, in a wheelchair insert or corner seat. Therapeutic positioning and comfortable seating are essential for purposes of evaluation and training, as they facilitate concentration for learning and reduce fatigue.

The purpose of the physical assessment is to determine an anatomic site at which a controlled behavior can become both functionally reliable and voluntary. This purposeful movement activates an interface (the means by which a user communicates with his device), which in turn acts upon the device (see section on interfaces).

A number of variables must be considered when evaluating the adequacy of a particular anatomic site (hand, head, foot, etc.). These factors are delineated in Table 7-1.

Because they are the most natural sites for interfacing with a device, the hands and fingers are generally assessed first in a physical evaluation. Children with neuromuscular disabilities who exhibit limited range of motion, inability to cross midline, or abnormal reflex patterns are often precluded from exercising certain manual movements.

Although the head is often considered as an interface site before other body parts, a thorough evaluation of hand, finger, and foot control is warranted. If a reliable control site can be discovered from among these body parts, then the head and eyes can remain unencumbered. In turn, this freedom from unnatural attachments, such as head and chin pointers, allows for more natural communication via eye gaze and facial expression, vital elements in human nonverbal communication.

The foot is often overlooked or underrated as an interface site. Not only can the foot often be reliably controlled, but it may also be trained to activate as many as 225 different switch positions by slight alterations of its orientation in space (Eulenberg, 1982). A seemingly unrefined foot movement may become quite purposeful by virtue of a simple modification in the foot's elevation or attitude.

When evaluation of the extremities fails to reveal reliable voluntary control, the head and neck must then be considered as possible interface sites. Assessment of these anatomic sites involves, as did the others, an evaluation of movement range, resolution and control, force and endurance.

Speech and Language
Cognitive Prerequisites to Language

Cognition is defined as the mediation and organization of thought, perceptions, and experiences, and the product of these processes. Our cognitive "stockpiles" increase as we experience meaningful interactions

Table 7-1
Factors to consider when evaluating accuracy of motion.

1.	*Range of Motion*	Maximal distance of body motion sweeping across the vertical and horizontal plane. Data are generally obtained from a zero reference point, the position at rest (Coleman, Cook, & Meyers, 1980).
2.	*Resolution of Motion*	Minimal movement that can be reliably and accurately executed (Coleman et al., 1980).
3.	*Force*	Amount of pressure exerted by a given body part.
		Measurement can be obtained by using a calibrated strain-gauge bridge (Coleman et al., 1980) or by using commercial switches that are pregauged and have a narrow range of adjustment capability.
4.	*Control*	Consistency and reliability of voluntary motion for a given body site.
		Data on speed, accuracy, and reliability of purposeful movement can be obtained by using a stop watch or establishing criteria trials.
		The presence of abnormal reflexes, spasticity, and tremors may compromise speed and accuracy, and require adjustment in switch location.
5.	*Endurance*	Duration of optimum level of functioning for a given body site, i.e., the length of time a child can execute a particular movement before fatigue occurs.

with our environment. These interactions occur through observation, and both mental and motoric manipulation of events, objects, and ideas. Normally developing children independently and frequently conduct these manipulations; handicapped children, due to physical and/or intellectual impairment, often cannot proceed beyond rudimentary cognitive levels without outside intervention.

The responsibility of the "interventionists"—parents, teachers, speech pathologists, and others—is to see that the child receives the greatest possible exposure to various environments, and, if necessary, to help him or her to see relationships and develop concepts. Many researchers believe that linguistic achievement depends on the acquisition of certain cognitive prerequisites, although their acquisition in and of itself is not the only determining factor (Bloom, 1970; Bowerman, 1974; Chapman & Miller, 1980; Cromer, 1974). Among the necessary prelinguistic processes are visual tracking and visual search, object permanence, means-end relationships, objective causality, imitation, functional classification of objects, functional object grouping, and seriation (Bricker & Bricker, 1974).

Although their conceptual development may be qualitatively different from normal acquisition, physically and/or mentally handicapped children are required to communicate with normal speakers using conventional language structure and strategies. Therefore, the child's level of proficiency in understanding and using "normal" language must be evaluated.

Prelinguistic abilities are actually cognitive abilities achieved as children interact with and, thereby, learn to understand their environment. These abilities may be evaluated by observing children in interaction with their surroundings, noting their expectancies and intentions, and monitoring the purposiveness of their actions. Their physical handicaps may require that the environment be modified to allow them to act upon it. For example, only after children begin to understand the causal relationships between themselves and their surroundings are they prepared to apply the concept of causality to language. They observe relationships between words and actions, and come to realize that actions or vocalizations effect an environmental change.

True linguistic operations include: "yes/no" responding; representation of objects, ideas, and feelings via vocalization, pictures, or more abstract symbols; and combinations of these representations into acceptable structures. Nonspeakers' abilities in these areas are evaluated by both conventional and nonconventional means.

A major consideration in naturalistic assessment is the child's preferred mode of response. By definition, the nonspeaker does not or cannot functionally utilize the oral musculature for verbal communication; therefore, responses must be channelled through other modalities. Evaluation of affirmation/negation ability may reveal a "yes" response to be a traditional head nod, or no more than a brief upward eye gaze. Regardless of the method used to communicate, the most important considerations are the consistency and appropriateness of the response.

The child's ability to identify objects and indicate choices can be evaluated by presenting him or her with an array of objects or pictures, and instructing the child to choose among them. Having determined the child's physical capabilities as well as limitations, the array may be modified to correspond to his or her response mode. This may necessitate transferring the display to an augmentative device.

In terms of production, the child functions at a holophrastic (one-word) level when he or she can consistently choose one item from an array. Expansion and diversification of the array's vocabulary permit word combinations, allowing the user to communicate with more grammatically advanced structures. Evaluation of the progression from one-word to multiword utterances involves manipulation of the number of selections presented, the various word classes, and the degree of complexity and abstractness of the representations.

These prelinguistic and linguistic categories are broad parameters of the speech/language assessment. More detailed information regarding specific areas may be gained through use of commercially available language-evaluation materials, again modifed to suit the child's response mode. Of equal importance is identification of those sensory channels most efficient and effective for each individual. With the accumulated information regarding the child's speech and language, physical and cognitive capabilities, the process of identifying appropriate augmentative systems continues.

Communication Systems

Augmentative communication refers to any system employed to enhance the communicative effectiveness of a message-sender. The system used may reflect the user's language or may introduce a new way of expressing ideas. The range of systems available for communication enhancement falls into three major categories: gestural systems, language boards, and electronic devices. These categories, as will be shown, are not mutually exclusive.

Providing the appropriate augmentative system involves much more than the introduction of a device. It also requires:

1. Determination of the appropriate semantic-transfer system;
2. Thorough instruction in the capabilities and limitations of the system;

3. Continued training and practice with the system; and

4. On-going re-evaluation of the system's effectiveness.

Gestural Systems

Gestural systems include manual sign languages, pantomine, yes/no indications, eye blink encoding, gestural Morse code, pointing, and other formalized and informal gesture systems (Silverman, 1980). Manual sign language systems, among which are Signed English, Standard, American Indian, American Sign Language, and Rochester systems, have continued to be applied as augmentative modes. The various systems differ in their iconicity and their similarity to the syntax of spoken English. To detail these variations would exceed the scope of this chapter; excellent references in this area include texts by Wilbur (1979) and Klima and Bellugi (1979). Silverman (1980) describes both the sign language systems and other gestural modes.

Manual sign language as an augmentative system is limited by the degree of physical coordination necessary for its use. Signs may be modified to require use of only one hand and to necessitate fewer discrete movements. These concessions notwithstanding, a major difficulty remains—gestures are effective as an expressive mode only as long as they are decoded correctly. The person relying solely on a gestural system will suffer from the effects of a pervasive language barrier in a real-world situation, not unlike the tourist in a foreign country whose knowledge of the native tongue is limited to words for "bathroom" and "How much is it?"

Language Boards

The second type of system involves use of language boards, which assume many forms and employ a wide variety of semantic-transfer systems. Language boards are usually two-dimensional arrangements of visually represented objects and ideas from which the user selects his choice. Language boards may be mounted on wheelchair trays or folders, attached to ambulation equipment or furniture, or worn on the user's body. On nonelectronic language boards, lexical choices are indicated primarily by direct selection; this, and other methods of selection will be discussed later in the chapter.

Language boards may employ a variety of semantic-transfer systems. "Semantic-transfer system" means a system for communicating meaning from a sender to a receiver. An all-encompassing term such as this is necessary for describing all levels of units found in a communication system.

A symbol, according to Silverman (1980), is a sensory (visual, auditory, or tactile) image, or sign, that suggests, or stands for, something else by reason of relationship (association) or convention. The most common symbols are our alphabet and number systems; despite their frequent use, they are among the most complex symbolic possibilities for use on a language board. More basic systems involve use of drawings at various levels of cognitive complexity. To clarify this issue, try the following exercise:

Read each statement and imagine the object or symbol described. See if you can visualize the progression from concrete to abstract.

A life-size red rose

A minature red rose

A full-size color photograph of a red rose

A scaled-down color photograph of a red rose

A colored line drawing of a red rose

A black and white drawing of a red rose

A stylized rendition of a red rose

What you just encountered was a hierarchical arrangement based on level of abstraction. Silverman (1980) states, "The *level of abstraction* of a picture is a function of the amount of detail (or information) present in the object or event depicted that is included in the picture. The more detail (or information) omitted, the higher the level of abstraction (p. 9)."

Level of abstraction is an important consideration when designing a board for a cognitively impaired person. The cognitive prerequisites to language discussed earlier are necessary for symbolization (allowing one unit to represent another). If this cognitive/linguistic milestone has not been reached, the child will not be able to conceptualize the derivation of the symbol from its referent. These same symbols may still be taught, yet in a remedial manner (Guess, Sailor, & Baer, 1974). In addition to the level of abstraction, it is necessary to consider other dimensions in the creation of a language board, including degree of complexity, degree of ambiguity, size, and the number of messages that can be encoded (Silverman, 1980).

By degree of complexity we mean the "busy-ness" of the symbol. For instance, a representation of "Mom" would be better expressed by a simple picture of the child's mother against a plain background than a picture of Mother, dressed in her Easter finery, posed with the family in front of a blossoming cherry tree.

The latter image is also useful in our illustration of degree of ambiguity; the photograph described could be used to represent Mom, family, springtime, Easter, standing, tree, and so on; in other words, it is ambiguous.

One aim in determining units for a language board is to reduce the degree of complexity. We concur with Silverman (1980) that "reducing complexity is one way of reducing ambiguity" (p. 90).

Picture size is a major consideration in designing a language board. Not only is size related to level of abstraction, but it is a crucial factor in regard to the user's visual abilities. Many small pictures grouped closely together necessitate not only finer visual discriminations, but also adequate figure-ground manipulation (i.e., singling out the desired picture from the background of the entire display).

It is also necessary to consider the number of messages that can be encoded with the chosen "vocabulary." Central to this determination are the child's level of functioning, and his environmental and educational needs. For the cognitively impaired, functional communication might best be facilitated by a language board picturing immediate environmental needs (cup, dish, toilet, etc). The more linguistically advanced will need to communicate basic needs as well as more complex ideas. One educational goal might be to foster correct sentence structure by the use of a language board. In this case, verbs and functor words would be included in the display.

Decisions regarding symbol inclusion are often difficult. Silverman (1980) suggests the following guideline: "The smallest set of pictures should be selected by which necessary messages can be encoded" (p. 90). McDonald and Schultz (1973) propose a complementary solution: The child should have different boards for different situations (home, classrooms, etc.).

The "rose" exercise presented earlier illustrated the levels of abstraction found in symbolic representation. Recall the most abstract version of the rose—of all the possibilities, this depiction has the least resemblance to the actual rose. It is this type of graphic representation that we shall next discuss.

Pictures are a very basic form of representation. Even more basic would be actual objects representing other objects (doll shoe for child's shoe). More complex than either of these options would be symbols that bear less, little, or no resemblance to their referents. This more complex type of symbol will first be generally addressed, and a review of some semantic-transfer systems currently in use for augmentative purposes will follow.

Symbols function at three levels of complexity, which have been described by Shane and Blau (1981). The first, in which the idea or object is clearly depicted at a concrete level, is known as the *pictographic*, or iconic level. Pictures and picture-like drawings fit into this category. A more complex level is the *ideographic*, or relational, symbol; in this case, the user must decipher the meaning from the symbol or combination of symbols presented to him. At this level, the symbol does not directly resemble its referent; however, prior explanation of the symbol's relation to the referent, or familiarity with the symbol's components, allows the user to derive meaning from it (see the Blissymbol examples that follow). The third level is the *arbitrary* level, at which the symbol has no discernible relationship to its referent. The written word is an example of this third level of complexity. These symbolic levels will become more clearly delineated as examples of each are encountered in the following discussion of symbol systems.

Blissymbolics is a symbol system originally devised for international, translinguistic communication by Charles Bliss (1965). Based on Chinese-type ideographic symbols, it is semantically based and relates to no specific language. Although Blissymbolics has not been widely accepted for its original purpose, it has found application as a semantic-transfer system for handicapped children (Archer, 1977; Carlson, 1976; Harris-Vanderheiden, 1976; Silverman, McNaughton & Kates, 1978), for it serves as a bridge between pictures and the written word.

The Blissymbol system contains approximately 100 basic symbols which, alone or in combination, can represent a surprisingly large number of ideas. In addition to representing objects and ideas, the symbols encode tense, inflection, and other grammatical indicators. Manipulation of the basic symbols along the dimensions of size, combination, and relative placement allow for almost limitless expression. All three levels of complexity (pictographic, ideographic, and arbitrary) are represented in this system.

     ○ represents "eye"

     ⊃ represents "ear"

     ⚡ represents "electricity"

     □ represents "thing"

Thus, combining them, □○⊃⚡ represents television, i.e., a thing run on electricity which we can see and hear.

Such symbols, when paired with various grammatical class indicators, take on different, yet related, meanings.

     □ denotes a noun

     ∧ denotes a verb

     ∨ denotes an adjective

     ⊃ represents "ear"

     ⊃̂ represents "to hear"

     ⊃̌ represents "auditory"

These isolated examples are not intended to provide a lesson in Blissymbolics, but rather to illustrate its fascinating workings. A summary of the system is provided by Silverman (1980), and the Blissymbolics Communication Institute (Toronto) publishes many materials, including the *Handbook of Blissymbolics for Instructors, Users, Parents and Administrators* (Silverman et al. 1978).

While Blissymbolics are international in nature, the Rebus system employs English vocabulary and phonology. Rebus symbols are primarily pictographic, but the pictures themselves are often combined with English phonemes or morphemes represented orthographically.

Rebuses are used to teach reading (Woodcock, 1958, 1965, 1968; Woodcock, Clark, & Davies, 1968, 1969) and facilitate language acquisition (Clark, Moores, & Woodcock, 1973), as well as serve as a semantic-transfer system on an augmentative device.

Another symbol system emerged from the Premacks' investigation of a chimpanzee's ability to learn human language (Premack, 1970, 1971; Premack & Premack, 1972, 1974). As the semantic-transfer system in these experiments, pieces of plastic, arbitrary in their design, were used. This system was applied to individuals who were unable to manipulate other types of linguistic units (Carrier & Peak, 1975). They developed the *Non-Speech Language Initiation Program (Non-SLIP)* to provide a "very carefully structured, finely graded, set of procedures for starting children through the process of learning communication skills" (Carrier & Peak, 1975, p. 10). Its primary use has been in teaching the basics of symbolic representation (Silverman, 1980).

As noted previously, alphabet and numbers are the semantic-transfer systems most apparent in our daily encounters. These systems may be represented in various configurations on a language board, such as:

1. an ordered alphanumeric line (A,B,C. . .and 1, 2, 3. . .);
2. placement based on frequency of occurrence; or
3. placement based on correspondence to the typewriter keyboard (referred to as "qwerty" in reference to the first six keys on the conventional keyboard's top alphabet row).

Morse code takes symbolization one step beyond the alphabet by requiring further symbolization of an already arbitrary system. Although Morse code can be represented visually (- . . , - . -), it is primarily an auditory system in which alphabet letters are encoded by sequences of long and short bursts of sound. Application of technology to augmentative systems has allowed Morse code to become a viable semantic-transfer system for handicapped users.

The symbol systems described previously are by no means the only ones in use on language boards. Items for inclusion on a board are often chosen from the child's personal lexicon. For example, pictures or drawings of the child's toys can be represented on the board in place of a generic representation of "toy." These familiar items are not only the most

FIGURE 7-1
Rebus symbols.

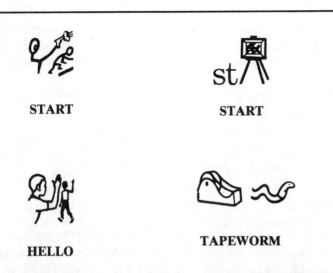

START	START
HELLO	TAPEWORM

meaningful for the child, but may also serve to ease the transition from one communication system to another.

Selection Modes

The use of electronic communication devices requires speech and language therapists to learn a few new terms and concepts if they are judiciously to choose the appropriate device for a given child. In this section, we will discuss these concepts, beginning with selection mode. "Selection mode" refers to the general means by which a user gets to (or "accesses") his semantic-transfer system. Thus, selection modes represent the various ways a child can access his vocabulary. The two types of selection modes are direct selection and scanning. The choice of one mode over the other depends on the child's physical and cognitive abilities; the primary difference between them is speed of communication.

The first of these modes, direct selection, is precisely that: the user directly indicates his chosen item on a display. Shane and Blau (1981) state that direct selection can be achieved by the use of:

1. an extremity (fist, elbow, finger, toe, etc.);
2. an extremity plus __ (splinted hand, hand-held pointer);
3. the eyes (directed gaze);

4. a rod (head or chin pointer, etc.); and

5. a light beam (mounted on body or held in hand or mouth).

Scanning is accomplished by halting a sequential presentation process when the desired choice is reached. Scanning is generally a slower and more complex mode of selection because the user must contend with the undesired choices as well as the desired ones.

Shane and Blau (1981) identified the various types of scanning as:

1. assisted scanning;

2. stepped scanning;

3. linear scanning;

4. row-column scanning; and

5. directed scanning.

Assisted scanning occurs when the user is required only to provide replies of the "affirmative/negative" type to a series of choices. A student at Pioneer Center uses this method to spell messages in the following way: (1) the child's communication partner determines if the message begins with a consonant or a vowel; (2) if it is a consonant, the child indicates in which half of the alphabet it occurs; and (3) letters are presented until the child indicates that his chosen letter has been reached with an upward eye movement indicating "yes."

The other four types of scanning are typically encountered when using electronic devices. At the risk of jumping ahead too quickly, Figure 7-2 shows a grid typical of those found on scanning devices to illustrate these other variations.

Stepped scanning requires the user to proceed one-at-a-time through the various selections. To reach the number 10 by stepped scanning, the user moves the indicator light (in the upper left corner of each cell) from 1 to 2, 2 to 3, and so on until he reaches 10. This requires 9 activations of the scanner.

Linear scanning also proceeds through all the selections before the desired one is reached, the difference being that it does not require an activation for each step. To access the number 10 requires 2 activations—one to begin the scan and one to stop it when it reaches the number 10. Although this method requires fewer activations, both the stepped and linear scanning methods share the drawback of the relatively long period of time required to scan every cell.

Row-column scanning somewhat alleviates this problem by scanning rows (on the horizontal axis) and columns (on the vertical axis), rather than individual cells. In this mode, all the lights in Row 1 glow first. The desired

FIGURE 7-2
Scanning device grid.

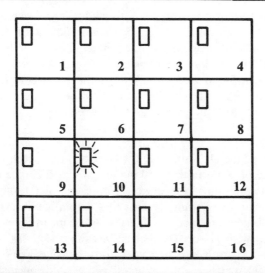

selection being in Row 3, the device continues scanning, next lighting up Row 2 and then Row 3, at which point the user indicates the row of choice by an activation of some kind. The device then begins scanning columns, proceeding from left to right. The scan stops at the second column, at which an activation lights up the number 10. This process requires three more activations than does linear scanning, yet is more efficient in terms of time.

Directed scanning occurs when the user communicates to the device the direction and amplitude of the scan. To access the number 10 in this mode, the user directs the device, using a joystick (the control stick similar to those found on many arcade games) to go over one column and down three rows. This requires more controlled movements on the part of the user, but markedly increases efficiency of communication. To further improve the rate of communication, these various scanning methods may be combined and modified in accordance with the user's needs.

Some approaches to nonspeech communication mention a third selection mode known as encoding. This technique employs coded information, selected either directly or by scanning, to access a larger lexicon. For instance, a student's language board may have expanded to include 500 items, yet the child lacks the range of motion necessary for direct selection over such a large area. As a solution, the rows may be labelled with alphabet letters and the columns with numbers, allowing the child to "encode" his choice by indicating the letter and number corresponding to his selection. Rather than consider encoding to be a third type of selection mode, we believe that it is more aptly termed a cognitive strategy (Shane & Blau, 1981), for it involves cognitive manipulation of predetermined codes, which are subsequently selected either directly or by scanning.

These selection modes—direct selection, scanning, and their related cognitive strategies—are the means by which the user accesses his semantic-transfer system. We will now turn our attention to the communication between the user and the device, and a new concept.

Interfaces

Knowledge of the child's physical, cognitive, and speech and language abilities is the prerequisite for making an informed choice regarding an augmentative communication device. The results of the physical assessment are particularly relevant, because they determine the type and placement of the chosen interface. An interface is the means by which the user communicates with his device, that is, how he makes his system work. Physically able persons use interfaces, too—consider remote-controlled televisions, light switches, and automatic garage-door openers. A requirement of all effective interfaces is that they be responsive to the capabilities of their user (Coleman et al., 1980). Figure 7-3 illustrates a variety of interfaces currently in use.

When choosing an interface, it is helpful to evaluate several switches at more than one anatomic site. The initial physical assessment serves as a good starting point, for it provides information as to the sites with most reliable control. Ongoing assessment of this type is also vital, because control may be trained and refined through practice. Evaluation of interfaces should entail quantification, as this allows for objective decision-making regarding final site/interface selection. Barker and Hastings (1981) suggest as the two major factors in this assessment, *tracking / select time* and *accuracy.* The first of these refers to the amount of time required for the user to move from a resting position to activation of the interface (tracking time), or from one aspect of the interface to another (select time). A temporal measurement in and of itself carries little meaning, unless it is accompanied by some indication of the appropriateness of the response; thus, an accuracy measure, when paired with a time measure, provides a more complete indication of the functionality of the site/interface match. It may be the case that one of these factors takes precedence over the other; for instance, when given the choice between a fast, yet inaccurate, interface site and a slower, more accurate one, the decision usually favors the latter option.

FIGURE 7-3
Zygo interfaces for "single switch" users.

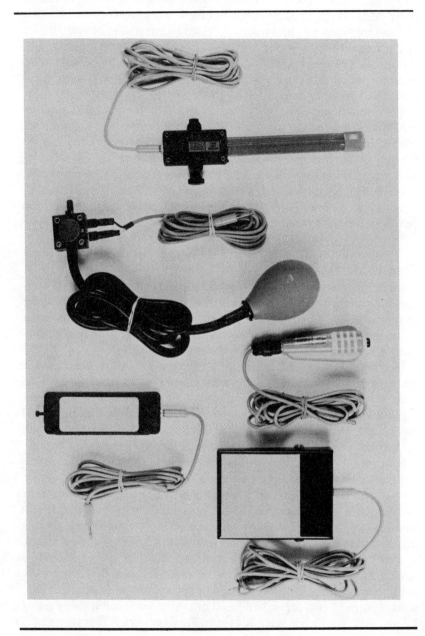

If one is to select an adequate interface, it is also important to consider the amount and type of feedback the child requires. Interfaces provide both environmental and performance feedback (Barker & Cook, 1981; Barker & Hastings, 1981). Environmental feedback is conducted through visual and auditory channels, and can be provided by buzzers, voice synthesizers, and any visual display (lights, LED or LCD characters, printout, etc.). Performance feedback includes tactile, proprioceptive, or kinesthetic information (Barker & Cook, 1981; Barker & Hastings, 1981), such as the amount of pressure needed for switch activation.

The primary factor in choosing an interface is the child's physical capabilities, but the key to effective interface positioning is experimentation. A slight variation in the switch's height or attitude (angle) may improve the user's effectiveness markedly. Although the process of experimenting with placement is somewhat serendipitous, the evaluation should not be; it is crucial to quantify the user's abilities (and preferences) along the dimensions discussed earlier—time and accuracy— in order to determine the most beneficial site/interface match.

Electronic Devices

Rather than attempt to review all devices currently available, this section will present a representative sample of commercial devices. The order of presentation follows the developmental hierarchy discussed previously in the speech and language evaluation section; the following devices augment prelinguistic as well as linguistic communication.

Electronic devices, such as signal boxes (similar to call-systems used in hospitals and on airplanes) and adapted toys (See Figure 7-4) serve the child at the prelinguisitc stage by allowing him to manipulate and effect his environment. "Yes/no" responses may be coded with an auditory signal box or by a device made expressly for this purpose. One such device, with both visual and auditory feedback, is pictured in Figure 7-5.

Following the progression introduced earlier, the next level of linguistic complexity involves choosing a selection from an array; this procedure is the basis for the introduction of language boards. Electronic devices may also serve as a sort of language board, displaying from only a few to several hundred selections. Converting a language board to an electronic display may decrease the motor requirements for selection and may provide visual, as well as auditory feedback. As with nonelectronic language boards, displays are primarily two-dimensional arrangements of lexical items. Electronic language boards have the additional options of scanning lights, printed output (hard copy), and taped or synthesized speech (See Figures 7-6 and 7-7). With a few exceptions (e.g., Prentke Romich Express systems

FIGURE 7-4
Toys.

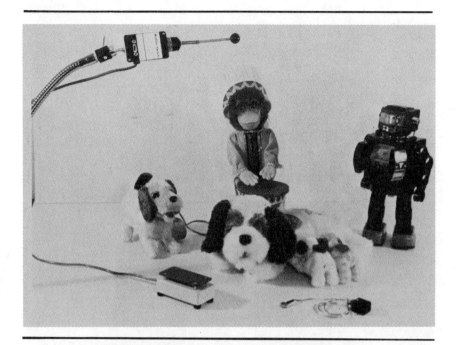

and Phonic Ear Vois 140), electronic language boards are designed to respond to only one selection mode, be it scanning or direct selection. These boards may employ any complexity level of semantic-transfer units, from photographs to words to the alphanumeric components of our language.

Keyboard instruments, on the other hand, rely strictly on alphanumeric characters for message coding. Modifications have been designed to accommodate the user's sensory and physical limitations. Keyboards are expanded (i.e., the keys are distributed over a larger area) to aid the person with poorly defined fine-motor movements; for those with limited range of motion, such as the inability to cross midline, keyboards may be reduced in size. Keyguards (see Figure 7-8) are designed for securing placement of the key selector (e.g., hand, chin, or head pointer). Figure 7-9 illustrates keyboards with liquid crystal (LCD) and light-emitting diode (LED) displays for providing visual feedback.

Microcomputers are another kind of keyboard instrument, but, unlike conventional keyboard devices, microprocessor-based systems have memory, storage, and programming capabilities. They may serve as aids for oral and

FIGURE 7-5
Zygo model 20 2-light choice indicator.

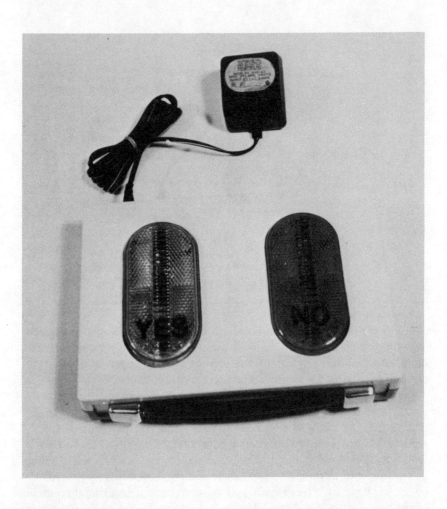

written communication, education, entertainment, and vocations. As with other systems, one of the primary problems our students encounter is that of access (interface) to the device. Resolution of access problems will

FIGURE 7-6
Zygo model 16 electronic communication system.

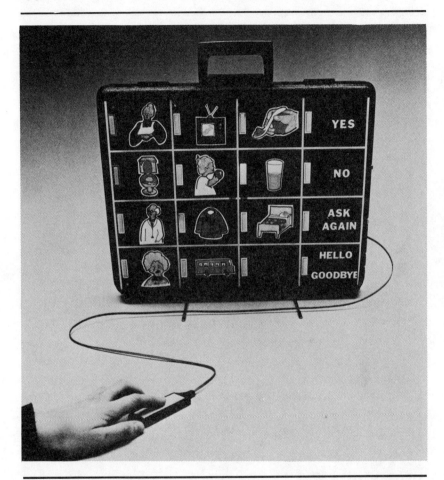

convert potential application of microprocessor-based systems into realities (Nelson et al., 1980).

The basic components of microcomputer devices are the hardware and software elements. "Hardware" refers to the actual machinery, i.e., the mechanical and electrical parts of the system. The significant part of the hardware is the silicon chip, smaller than a fingernail, which controls the "software" by completing the instruction of the software specifies. Thus, the software component refers simply to a set of instructions to make the machinery respond to the user's directives. The following paragraphs will

FIGURE 7-7
Zygo model 100 with model 2016 — display/printer.

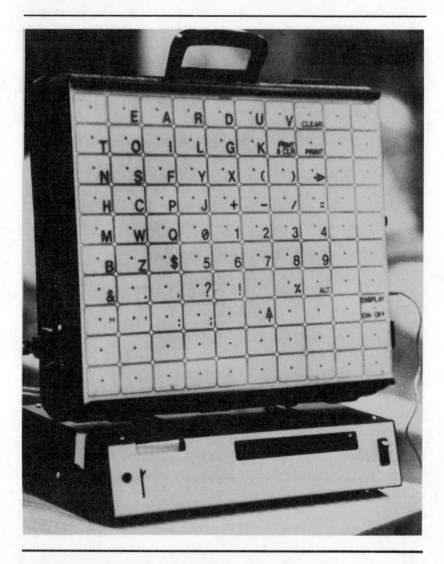

address two types of microcomputer devices as these systems apply to nonspeaking physically handicapped children.

Figure 7-10 illustrates the type of microprocessor-based devices which have preprogrammed lexicons of phrases, letters and phonemes. These

FIGURE 7-8
Canon Communicator with keyguard.

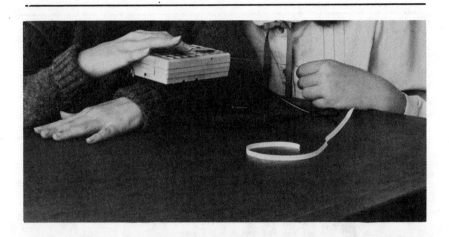

portable systems have memory capability, visual display (LED and LCD), and offer vocal and/or hard copy (printed) output. The devices shown in Figures 7-10 through 7-12 illustrate instruments that have preprogrammed lexicons, as well as capability to allow the user to program a personalized vocabulary, to control environmental operations of powered wheelchairs, appliances, lights, radios, tape recorders, etc., to select printed versus visual versus vocal output, and to interconnect to a general-purpose computer. The Semantically Accessible Language Board (SAL) displayed in Figure 7-12 utilizes the basic elements of other systems previously mentioned, with additional software components such as "text-to-speech" capability. This allows for a synthetic speech production of a printed input; for example, selection of the keys C-H-R-I-S results in the synthesized articulation of "Chris."

Some students are able to use ready-made over-the-counter general purpose microcomputers rather than customized instruments. These popular systems, such as the Apple and TRS-80, are flexible, "portable," and moderately prices in a highly competitive market, and offer increased availability of educational and recreational software. Several manufacturers have so miniaturized the entire microcomputer system that "pocket" computers are now readily available and affordable. These small versions permit increased portability, while retaining the majority of the features of their larger counterparts.

FIGURE 7-9
Sharp Memowriter and VIP Communicator.

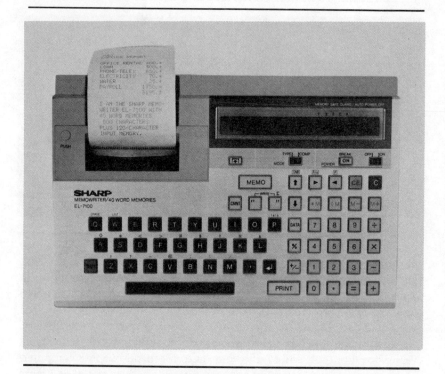

Some general examples of microcomputer applications are:
1. storage and retrieval of information;
2. text editing of oral annd written communication;
3. composition of oral and written communication;
4. operation of common environmental appliances; and
5. provision of computer-assisted instruction for educational, vocational, and personal purposes (Rogers, Fine, Kuhlemeir, & Bowen, 1980).

Although microcomputers are traditionally direct-selection devices, minimal hardware and/or software modifications render these devices responsive to scanning techniques and encoded input (Morse code, etc.). A microcomputer's inherent flexibility enables the device to be modified as the user's physical and cognitive skills develop beyond the scope of his current system (Heckathorne, Doubler, & Childress, 1980).

FIGURE 7-10
Phonic Ear Vois 130 and Phonic Ear Vois 140.

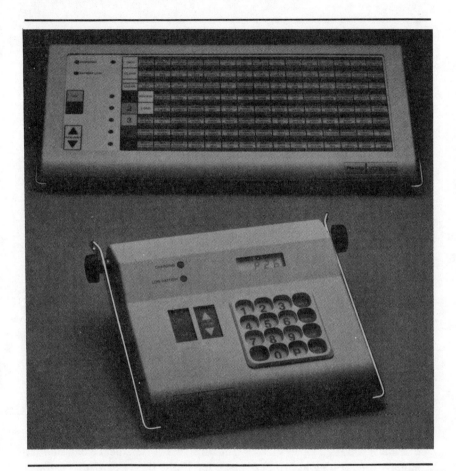

Case Histories

We have previously charted the course to follow when matching an augmentative device to a nonspeaker's needs. The procedure entails first assessing the child's abilities, the device's or system's capability, and then employing this information to interface the child to the device. To better illustrate this process, case histories of three children are pertinent. All of the students attend Pioneer Center and have been mentioned earlier in this chapter.

FIGURE 7-11
Prentke Romich Express 3.

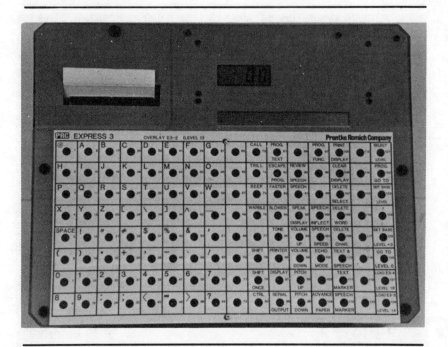

Diana (10 years old) is severely cerebral-palsied, visually impaired and mentally retarded. Her extreme physical disability prohibits not only functional oral communication, but also fine motor coordination. Gross motor movements are characterized by extension and spasticity. Results obtained from structured observations and informal assessment suggest that Diana is functioning at a prelinguistic level. She does not visually track, and is only now achieving the concept of causality. Although she sometimes indicates affirmation by an "eyes up" motion, this response is not consistent.

Physical assessment suggests that getting Diana interfaced to a simple switch is a difficult task, as she exhibits little reliable voluntary movement. Various anatomic sites and switches have been considered, and, at the present time, she is using a tread switch with performance and environmental feedback at her hand to access a tape recorder and toys. Seating modifications designed to minimize the effects of her spasticity include securing her in a corner seat to maintain midline arm postures and shoulder

FIGURE 7-12
Semantically Accessible Language (SAL) board.

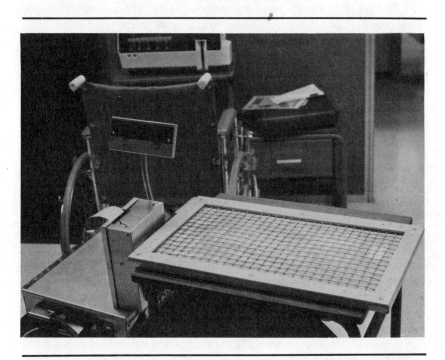

alignments, supporting her trunk with a vest, and stabilizing her free arm. Afforded opportunities to explore the function of the switch, Diana observed that its activation resulted in a pleasurable event (hearing music or voices on tape). Through repeated practice, she has begun to establish a cause-and-effect relationship between these two events. Establishment of this relationship is a vital step on the language acquisition hierarchy.

Janice (age 14), on the other hand, has progressed beyond prelinguistic behaviors to meaningful use of a limited number of language units. She has many physical problems (repaired cleft palate, Down's syndrome, arthrogryposis); until recently, her physical problems precluded walking. However, her hands and oral structures are physically capable of the activity necessary for communication. The hindrance to language development is Janice's low cognitive ability, but her increasing age makes the need for a functional method of communication all the more urgent.

Janice lacks the motivation to learn language because she seems to be unaware of the power that language wields. Therapeutic goals focus on providing Janice with a taste of communication's potency in the belief that once she experiences it, language will become naturally reinforcing.

To this end, Janice was first introduced to different augmentative devices in the hope that their novelty would spark interest and experimentation. A language board "notebook" was provided as well as a language board on her walker; a simple scanner and an eye-gaze system were also introduced. Janice's interest in these systems was short-lived, possibly because she failed to comprehend the communicative potential of her new "toys."

Attention was redirected to Janice's own communicators—her hands and mouth. Her language at this point was primarily nonfunctional, comprised of unrefined gestures, babbling, and some sterotypical phrases. Efforts were concentrated on helping Janice to see that her behaviors could exert control over her world. To this end, manual signs representing functional concepts such as "open, " "put in, " and "sleep" were modeled, shaped, prompted, and reinforced. This approach has proven successful and continues to be implemented in Janice's communication program.

Jennifer (13 years old) is extremely motivated and independently "explores" strategies to augment her communication. She is severely physically impaired due to cerebral palsy and requires total assistance for basic living functions. Although spelling and comprehension of spoken language are appropriate for her age and grade level, her academic performance in reading and arithmetic is not.

Physical assessment revealed the absence of any natural voluntary hand or foot movement for executing purposeful control. Seated and posture-stabilized, Jennifer directly accessed language boards and keyboard devices. Her experiences with these systems—Micon, HandiVoice 120 and typewriter keyboard—were at best frustrating compromises. Speed and accuracy, necessary in interaction, were virtually nonexistent.

Preferring to have her eyes and head free to explore her world, Jennifer refused to use obtrusive head or chin pointers, as well as electronic scanning instruments. However, her positive experiences with an unobtrusive small headlight pointer modified these attitudes. Available on her wheelchair tray is a 7×6 language board matrix displaying the alphabet, key words, phrases, and syllables. Her transmission of information is presently limited by her receiver's abilities to read and synthesize the selections at her rate of output, and the absence of voice and paper printout.

Currently these problems are tentatively resolved. Using a microcomputer with a customized interface which accepts the headlight input, Jennifer generates and transmits information. The continued availability of the relatively inexpensive microcomputer instruments will provide Jennifer educational, recreational, and vocational opportunities.

Recent Trends

Hardware

The gap between nonspeakers and their vocal counterparts has narrowed in the past decade, due to the application of technology in the area of augmentative communication. Unfortunately, most nonspeech communication continues to lack the speed and flexibility of normal interactions. Clinical applications have indicated that the most efficient and effective means of alleviating this problem is not through introduction of individual customized devices, but through modifications to readily available general purpose computers (GPCs), such as those made by Radio Shack, Atari, Apple, and Texas Instruments.

One GPC may now, by virtue of software and interface options, subsume the role of myriad customized devices. The same unit may serve as a keyboard device, an environmental control system, a scanner, a call system, a printer, and a voice synthesizer. The trend indicates that pocket computers will offer the full capabilities of a microcomputer.

The approach to interfacing is moving toward utilizing more natural movements in the control of devices, and away from requiring the user to adapt to contrived environments. For example, harnessing the voluntary control of Jennifer's head to direct a lightbeam is much less intrusive than subjecting her to an unnatural arm posture for the purpose of accessing a keyboard.

Tapping the intact abilities of nonspeakers is the most natural interfacing strategy. Such vital bodily activities as eye gaze, blood flow, muscular contraction, and even brain waves can be trained through biofeedback techniques to become reliable means by which to control a device (Beal, 1982). Even nonspeech vocal productions may be shaped and employed as a control mode.

Although there are many techniques for monitoring eye gaze, all are based on the observation that eye movement capabilities are generally intact in cerebral-palsied persons (Anderson, 1977; Fincke & O'Leary, 1980). One method used to determine eye position picks up electrical signals from the eye muscles that are amplified, filtered, interpreted and then mediated through a microcomputer for the purpose of controlling various devices (Laefsky & Roemer, 1978).

Other systems monitor eye gaze by detecting the corneal reflection of an infrared light source (Fincke & O'Leary, 1980; Rinard & Rugg, 1978; Rosen & Durkee, 1978). These systems contain computers that determine where the user is looking, relative to a display, by employing data from eye direction and, in some cases, from orientation of the head as determined by ultrasonography.

Other systems employ eye gaze as a sort of joystick control, requiring the user to gaze in one of several specific directions. Combinations of these signals designate various alphanumeric, punctuation, and control symbols via a coded input (Rosen & Durkee, 1978).

Speech recognition is the process by which a microprocessor is controlled through spoken input. Only ten years ago scientists predicted that this century would not see sophisticated applications of the speech-recognition technique (Doddington & Schalk, 1981); 1980s' technology has already proven them wrong. Not only can our machines talk to us via synthetic speech, but we can control them via verbal requests. Voice data entry becomes necessary when: (1) other body parts are occupied or otherwise unable to input data; and (2) the task requires mobility, thereby precluding stationary communication with the computer.

To commend speech recognition as an interface method for nonspeakers seems paradoxical, yet one must bear in mind that a nonspeaker is one for whom speech is a nonfunctional communication mode. This is not to say that a nonspeaker has no vocal output; rather, that his or her vocal productions are generally unintelligible and therefore not useful in reciprocal speech systems.

Speech recognition systems for the functional nonspeaker are programmed to be responsive to whatever consistent vocalizations the user produces. These may range from unintelligible renditions of words to single vowel productions; however, regardless of the level of complexity of production, the vocalization must be consistent to enable the computer to recognize the features by which intentions are classified. As Doddington and Schalk (1981) commented, "Consistency is an elusive goal," and not a problem limited solely to the speaker. Changes in the environment (affecting noise and reverberation) and in microphone placement can contribute to inconsistency (Doddington & Schalk, 1981). These problems are at present being addressed by research (Eulenberg, 1982).

As we attempt to utilize more natural movement in interfacing, the trend is toward maximizing the information that can be gained by a single input, thus minimizing the energy required. Whereas a single switch traditionally permits an all-or-nothing, on/off choice, proportional control allows for gradations of switch inputs. Although proportionally controlled interface systems are primarily used for the operation of wheelchairs, these same principles are being applied to communication devices as well.

Software

Employing innovative interfacing techniques is not the only means by which to make a general purpose computer (GPC) compatible with a user's needs; software design can further simplify and systematize communication via computer. A GPC's greatest attribute is its ability to store and retrieve tremendous amounts of information. When this capacity is fully exploited, the system demands some sort of organizational network to make information retrieval more efficient. This is especially relevant for the physically handicapped user who cannot afford to expend energy in numerous key selections.

Innovative software design is the solution to this problem. One general approach involves revising programs designed to be accessed directly, by making them responsive to selection by scanning. In this way, the user need only input signals to direct the scanning, rather than expend several keystrokes in typing a message. Other software changes may rearrange and/or systematize the information to make selection more efficient. Three examples of these specific modifications to software—chunking, predictive scanning, and layered hierarchies—are detailed below.

The chunking system, developed by Goodenough-Trepagnier and Prather (1979), and based on traditional orthography, employs phoneme sequences, as well as individual alphabet letters, in its semantic transfer system. The sequences were chosen in terms of frequency of occurrence in English, and require the user to activate fewer selections than would be necessary in a purely single-character system. Chunking has application not only to microcomputers (Goodenough-Trepagnier, Goldenburg, & Fried-Oken, 1981) but to nonelectronic language boards as well. Including more phoneme sequences on the display reduces the selection gestures, thus increasing communication rate (Goodenough-Trepagnier & Prather, 1981).

Another time- and effort-saving software design involves prediction of subsequent units from those previously entered. Prediction of this sort works at all linguistic levels—phonetic, morphological, syntactic, and semantic. It is in essence a "most likely to succeed" guessing game, in that the computer decides what letter is most likely to succeed the input "T R E" (Lee, 1982) or what word is most likely to complete the phrases, "The squirrel ran up the __ ." Some programs are designed to expand telegraphic sentences; for instance, the user would input "I go home", and the computer would produce "I am going home" (Hillinger, Fox, & Wilson, 1981).

Predictive scanning was introduced as a solution to the often tedious nature of row-column scanning. In this latter method, the user must wait until his selection is approached by the scanner and has no means by which to "skip over" the undesired selections. Predictive scanning's "dynamic matrix" changes the actual configuration of the letters so that the ones "most likely to succeed" are the easiest and fastest to access (Jones, 1981).

The use of predictive scanning has increased communication speed from 200% to 400% (Jones, 1981).

The final software design method to be discussed is that of hierarchical arrangements of information. These layered hierarchies, or menus, are arranged so that the information contained becomes increasingly specific as the progression through them continues. For instance:

Selecting VERBS from the main menu yields a menu of verbs in the infinitive form; selection of one of these infinitives yields a sub-menu—a list of conjugations of that verb. When one of these is selected, it is appended to a message. Theoretically, a word list could contain menus to an arbitary degree; however, in practial use, there has never been a need for more than 3 layers of menu (Buus, 1981, p. 132).

Menus may also be based on alphabetization, word frequency, or situational constraints (Campbell and Nieves, 1981).

Permutations and Combinations

Systematic Evaluation

Computers, previously discussed as instructional and communication devices, may also assist in the systematic assessment of a child's abilities. Not only has software been designed to evaluate cognitive and perceptual abilities, but microprocessor-based systems have been devised to evaluate the child's capacity for device control.

Barker and colleagues developed a control evaluator and trainer kit to assess anatomic sites systematically (Barker & Cook, 1981; Barker & Hastings, 1981). The Barker system, a portable self-contained microprocessor-based evaluation-and-training device, uses performance and environmental feedback to facilitate quantitative measurements of control. Anatomic sites are ranked in terms of the user's ability to exercise purposeful movement or the range over which voluntary control can be effectively exercised (Barker & Cook, 1981; Barker & Hastings, 1981).

Firmware

The need for hardware and/or software modifications decreases the number of commercial computer programs available to physically disabled individuals. Further, adaptations can be exorbitantly expensive simply because these programs are not easily changed. At the University of Washington and at the Trace Center-University of Wisconsin a technique that uses an adaptive-firmware card has been developed for the Apple II.

The firmware card allows the disabled client to use standard commercial software without the expense of hardware and/or software modifications. Thus, a vast library of commercial programs becomes readily available to the user.

The adaptive-firmware card makes the computer think that the keyboard is actually providing the input. The insertion of the card into the microcomputer provides a variety of "transparent" inputs, including scanning, Morse code, and direct selection (Schwejda & Vanderheiden, 1982). These inputs are referred to as "transparent" because they work in conjunction with other programs, without requiring that these programs be altered in any way. The keyboard input can come from a variety of interfaces, such as single-switch, dual switches, joysticks, or paddle controls.

Another technique currently being investigated at the Trace Center-University of Wisconsin is the design of universal keyboard emulators to work with a variety of personal computers and terminals. The keyboard emulators not only mimic the actual keyboard of the computer, but are also invisible to the system. The microcomputer is deceived into thinking the message originated from direct keyboard input, rather than through an emulator. With the emulator installed, normal use of the computer keyboard can continue. The application of this technique will allow handicapped clients to use nonstandard input devices such as communication aids or other micro and hand-held computers.

Hybrid Lightbeam/Sensor Technique

The combination of two types of head/light-pointing techniques has resulted in the improved "hybrid light" developed at the Trace Center-University of Wisconsin (Vanderheiden, 1982a, 1982b, 1982c). This new selection device has as its ancestor the humble headstick, a simple wand attached to the head by means of a hat-like contraption. It allows the user to directly select elements from a language board. The headstick, like all other devices, has both benefits and drawbacks. The benefit is that the head can be one of the body parts with the most precise voluntary movement. A very obvious drawback is the unnatural appearance and cumbersome handling of the large apparatus.

A selection mechanism using lights need not be large and cumbersome, yet it should allow the user to take advantage of good voluntary head control. These considerations prompted development of two types of electronic headsticks in use today.

The first is simply a lightbeam-emitting device akin to a tiny flashlight mounted on a band around the user's head. This allows the user to direct the light beam onto whatever he intends to indicate, which may be not only selections on a language board, but also choices among foods in a meal, people in a room, or various toys. The benefit of this system is the constant visual feedback provided by the lightbeams regarding head position. The drawback, at the present time, is the unavailability of a commercial system responsive to this type of light input.

The other type of device employs a photoreceptive sensor, rather than an actual light in the head-mounted apparatus. This is then used in conjunction with a discrete LED device, such as the Express III (see Figure 7-11). Behind each selection block on the face of the device is a small LED. When the user centers the light-sensitive receptor worn on the head over this spot, the message is relayed to the device, and that unit is thus selected. The drawback of this system is that the "sweet spot" for selection is very small, and only when the user can center the sensor over the spot for the designated time is the selection accomplished. The device gives no visual feedback as to location of the sensor, simply an all-or-nothing activation of the individual LEDs.

The Trace Center's "hybrid light" is a combination of devices; it contains both the photoreceptive sensor and the lightbeam device. The photoreceptor works as before, allowing communication with a device for printing, display, and storage of the message; the addition of the lightbeam allows the user to constantly monitor his or her head positions, correcting minor excursions from the "sweet spot" with relative ease. In addition, the lightbeam may be used for selection in the absence of the user's electronic communication system.

Summary

The handicapped population benefits from our society's technological advances. Granted, not every nonspeaker can take advantage of highly sophisticated computers, nor can applications of technology solve every problem and overcome every limitation. In the hands of knowledgeable professionals, however, these new devices and systems can change lives.

In this discipline the human factor, rather than the machine, is the critical component. Employing information from assessments of both physical and cognitive functioning, professionals determine the status and needs of the nonspeaker. Knowledge of available systems and interfacing techniques allows the professional to match the user with appropriate devices.

Even if this "matchmaking" is successful, it should never be the end of the line. Communication enhancement is not an event; it is a process. We revise our prescriptions as our clients change and grow, as we learn more, and—last, but not least—as technology continues to advance.

References

Anderson, K.E. An eye-position controlled typewriter. *Proceedings of the Workshop on Communication Aids for the Non-Verbal Physically Handicapped,* June 1977, 137-141.

Archer, L. Blissymobolics—A non-verbal communication system. *Journal of Speech and Hearing Disorders,* 1977, *42,* 568-579.

Barker, M.R., & Cook, A.M. A systematic approach to evaluating physical ability for control of assistive devices. *Proceedings of the Fourth Annual Conference on Rehabilitation Engineering,* 1981, 287-289.

Barker, M.R., & Hastings, W.R. Control evaluator and trainer kit. *Proceedings of the Johns Hopkins First National Search for Applications of Personal Computing to Aid the Handicapped,* 1981, 175-177.

Beal, J. Mind to mind communication. In Communications and the future, panel presented at Meeting of the World Future Society's Fourth General Assembly, Washington, D.C., 1982.

Bliss, C.K. *Semantography (Blissymbolics)* (2nd ed.). Sydney, Aus.: Semantography (Blissymbolics) Publications, 1965.

Bloom, L. *Language development: Structure and function in emerging grammars.* Cambridge, Mass. MIT Press, 1970.

Bowerman, M. Discussion summary—development of concepts underlying language. In R.L. Schiefelbusch & L.L. Lloyd (Eds.), *Language perspectives—Acquisition, retardation and intervention.* Baltimore: University Park Press, 1974.

Bricker, W.A., & Bricker, D.D. An early language training strategy. In R.L. Schiefelbusch & L.L. Lloyd, (Eds.), *Language perspectives—Acquisition, retardation and intervention.* Baltimore: University Park Press, 1974.

Buus, R. A computer communication aid for the nonverbal handicapped. *Proceedings of the Johns Hopkins First National Search for Applications of Personal Computing to Aid the Handicapped,* 1981, 131-135.

Campbell, R.S., & Nieves, L.A. Communication and environmental control system. *Proceedings of the Johns Hopkins First National Search for Application of Personal Computing to Aid the Handicapped,* 1981, 114-115.

Carlson, F.L. *An adapted communication project for a nonspeaking child.* Paper presented at the 51st Annual Convention of the American Speech and Hearing Association, Houston, November 1976.

Carrier, J.K., Jr., & Peak, T. *Program Manual for Non-SLIP (Non-Speech Language Initiation Program).* Lawrence, KS: H & H Enterprises, Inc., 1975.

Chapman, R.S., & Miller, J.F. Analyzing language and communication in the child. In R.L. Schiefelbusch (Ed.), *Nonspeech language and communication: Analysis and intervention.* Baltimore: University Park Press, 1980.

Clark, C.R., Moores, D.F., & Woodcock, R.W. *Minnesota Early Language Development Sequence.* Minneapolis: Research, Development & Demonstration Center in Education of Handicapped Children, University of Minnesota, 1973.

Coleman, C.L., Cook, A.M. & Meyers, L.S. Assessing non-oral clients for assistive communication devices. *Journal of Speech and Hearing Disorders,* 1980, *45,* 515-526.

Cromer, R.F. The development of language and cognition: The cognition hypothesis. In D. Foss (Ed.), *New perspectives in child development.* Baltimore: Penguin, 1974.

Cromer, R.F. The cognitive hypothesis of language acquisition and its implications for child language deficiency. In D. Morehead & A. Morehead (Eds.), *Normal and deficient child language.* Baltimore: University Park Press, 1976.

Doddington, G.R., & Schalk, T.B. Speech recognition: Turning theory to practice. *IEEE Spectrum,* September 1981, *18,* 26-32.

Eulenberg, J. Personal communication, February 18, 1982.

Eulenberg, J. Personal communication, July 19, 1982.

Fincke, R. & O'Leary, J.P., Jr. The design of a line of gaze interface for communication and environment manipulation. *Proceedings of the International Conference on Rehabilitation Engineering,* 1980, 96-97.

Goodenough-Trepagnier, C., Goldenburg, E.P., & Fried-Oken, M. Nonvocal communication system with unlimited vocabulary using Apple and SPEEC Syllables. *Proceedings of the Fourth Annual Conference on Rehabilitation Engineering,* 1981, 173-175.

Goodenough-Trepagnier, C., & Prather, P. *Manual for teachers of SPEEC.* Boston: Tufts-New England Medical Center, 1979.

Goodenough-Trepagnier, C., & Prather, P. Communication systems for the nonvocal based on frequent phoneme sequences. *Journal of Speech and Hearing Research,* 1981, *24,* (3), 322-329.

Guess, D., Sailor, W., & Baer, D.M. To teach language to retarded children. In R.L. Schiefelbusch & L.L. Lloyd (Eds.), *Language perspectives—Acquisition, retardation and intervention.* Baltimore: University Park Press, 1974.

Harris, D., & Vanderheiden, G. Enhancing the development of communicative interaction. In R.L. Schiefelbusch (Ed.), *Nonspeech language and communication: Analysis and intervention.* Baltimore: University Park Press, 1980.

Harris-Vanderheiden, D. Blissymbolics and the mentally retarded. In G.C. Vanderheiden & K. Grilley (Eds.), *Non-vocal communication techniques and aids for the severely physically handicapped.* Baltimore: University Park Press, 1976.

Heckathorne, C.W., Doubler, J.A., & Childress, D.S. Experiences with microprocessor-based aids for disabled people. *Proceedings of the Johns Hopkins First National Search for Applications of Personal Computing to Aid the Handicapped,* 1981, 53-56.

Hillinger, M., Fox, B., & Wilson, M. Computer-enhanced communication systems for the Apple II. *Proceedings of the Johns Hopkins First National Search for Applications of Personal Computing to Aid the Handicapped,* 1981, 16-18.

Jones, Randal L. Row/column scanning with a dynamic matrix. *Proceedings of the Johns Hopkins First National Search for Applications of Personal Computing to Aid the Handicapped,* 1981, 6-8.

Klima, E., & Bellugi, U. *The signs of language.* Cambridge, MA: Harvard University Press, 1979.

Laefsky, I.M., & Roemer, R.A. A real-time control system for CAI and prothesis. *Behavioral Research Methods and Instrumentation,* 1978, *10,* (2), 182-185.

Lee, S.A. A microcomputer-based VOCA for the non-vocal. *Proceedings of the Fifth Annual Conference on Rehabilitation Engineering,* 1982, 141-143.

McDonald, E.T., & Schultz, A.R. Communication boards for cerebral palsied children. *Journal of Speech and Hearing Disorders,* 1973, *38,* 73-88.

Morris, S.E. Communication/interaction development at mealtimes for the multiply handicapped child: Implication for the use of augmentative communication systems. *Language Speech and Hearing Services in Schools,* 1981, *12* (4), 216-232.

Nelson, D.J., Park, G.C., Farley, R.L., & Cote-Baldwin, C. Providing access to computers for physically handicapped persons: Two approaches. *Proceedings of the Fourth Annual Conference on Rehabilitation Engineering,* 1981, 140-142.

Non-speech communication: A position paper. *Asha,* 1980, *22* (4), 267-272.

Premack, A.J., & Premack, D. Teaching language to an ape. *Scientific American,* 1972, *277,* 92-99.

Premack, D. A functional analysis of language. *Journal of Experimental Analysis of Behavior,* 1970, *14,* 107-125.

Premack, D. Language in chimpanzee? *Science,* 1971, *172,* 808-822.

Premack, D., & Premack, A.J. Teaching visual language to apes and language deficient persons. In R.L. Schiefelbusch & L.L. Lloyd (Eds.), *Language perspectives—Acquisition, retardation and intervention.* Baltimore: University Park Press, 1974.

Rinard, G., & Rugg, D. Application of the ocular transducer to the ETRAN communicator. Conference on Systems and Devices for the Disabled, Houston, 1978.

Rinard, G., & Rugg, D. Communication/control application of the ocular transducer (Technical note 78-001), Denver Research Institute, University of Denver.

Rogers, J.T., Fine, P.R., Kuhlemeir, K.V., & Bowen, R.L. C2E2: A micro-computer system to aid the severely physically disabled in activities of daily living. *Proceedings of the International Conference on Rehabilitation Engineering,* 1980, 36-38.

Rosen, M.J., & Durkee, W.K. Preliminary report on EYECOM. Conference on Systems and Devices for the Disabled, Houston, 1978.

Schiefelbusch, R.L., & Hollis, J.H. A general system for nonspeech language. In R.L. Schiefelbusch (Ed.), *Nonspeech language and communication: Analysis and intervention.* Baltimore: University Park Press, 1980.

Schwejda, P., & Vanderheiden, G.C. Adaptive-firmware card for the Apple II. *Byte,* September 1982, *7* (9), 276-314.

Shane, H., & Blau, A. Paper presented at the Northeast Regional Conference of the American Speech and Hearing Association, July 1981.

Silverman, F.H. *Communication for the speechless.* Englewood Cliffs, NJ: Prentice-Hall, 1980.

Silverman, H., McNaughton, S., & Kates, B. *Handbook of Blissymbolics for instructors, users, parents and administrators.* Toronto: Blissymbolics Communication Institute, 1978.

Vanderheiden, G.C. Hybrid optical headpointing technique. *Proceedings of the Fifth Annual Conference on Rehabilitation Engineering,* 1982, 24. (a)

Vanderheiden, G.C. Lightbeam headpointer research. *Communication Outlook,* 1982, *4,* 11. (b)

Vanderheiden, G.C. Trace-hybrid lightbeam/sensor techniques. *Communication Outlook,* 1982, *3,* 6-7. (c)

Weiss, L. Personal communication, February 5, 1982.

Wilbur, R.B. *American sign language and sign systems.* Baltimore: University Park Press, 1979.

Woodcock, R.W. An experimental test for remedial readers. *Journal of Educational Psychology,* 1958, *49,* 23-27.

Woodcock, R.W. (Ed.) *The rebus reading series.* Nashville, TN: Institute on Mental Retardation & Intellectual Development, George Peabody College, 1965.

Woodcock, R.W. Rebuses as a medium in beginning reading instruction. *IMRID Papers and Reports,* 1968, *5* (4).

Woodcock, R.W., Clark, C.R., & Davis, C.O. *The Peabody rebus reading program.* Circle Pines, MN: American Guidance Service, 1968.

Woodcock, R.W., Clark, C.R., & Davies, C.O. *The Peabody Rebus Reading Program-Teacher's Guide.* Circle Pines, MN: American Guidance Service, 1969.

AUTHOR INDEX

SUBJECT INDEX

A

Achievement tests
  adolescent problems, 167
  California Achievement Test, 163
  Metropolitan Achievement Tests, 163
  Peabody Individualized Achievement Tests, 163
  Wide Range Achievement Tests, 163
Acquired aphasia, convulsive disorders
  assessment protocol, 71-72
  audiological characteristics, 64
  auditory verbal agnosia, 74-76
  behavioral characteristics, 64
  cognitive characteristics, 64
  communication breakdowns, 83, 92-97
  comparative data, *80-81*
  defined, 57
  EEG disturbances, 58, 67-69
  etiologies, 57
  evaluation, 71
  filled pauses, 83, 92-93
  grammatical marker usage, 93
  intervention, 58, 97
  language characteristics, *65, 70-71*
  language samples, 79
  learning-disabled data, 82
  male vs. female, 59-61
  mean length of utterance (MLU), 79, 84-87
  muteness, 65
  narrative vs. conversational samples, 83
  neurological characteristics, 59
  onset, 58-61
  pathogeneses, 67-69
  pilot data, 72-77
  prognosis, 58, 69-70
  research, 58-59, 70, 97
  similarities to learning-disabled, 93
  syntactic reformations, 93
  Systematic Analysis of Language Transcripts (SALT), 78
  utterance types, 83, 88-91
  vs. developmental, 73-74
  vs. learning-disabled, 77-97
  voice quality, 65
  word/phrase revision, 83, 93
  word retrieval problems, 93
Acquisition, normal language
  adult-child interaction, 105-108 (*see also* Maternal speech)
  age norms, 50-51
  & cognitive abilities, *52, 151-152*
  assessment, 49-53, 153 (*see also* Assessment)
  Brown's stages, 50-51
  causal relations, 24-25
  cohesive devices, 27-29
  communicative competence, 102, 108
  communicative functions, 5-7, *8-10,* 11, 26-27
  complex sentences, 23-26
  comprehension, 2-4, 11-12, 29-30
  contingent speech, 17-19
  conversational turn-taking, 20-21
  environmental influences, 47, 114 (*see also* Environmental influences)
  feedback, effects of, 105-108 (*see also* Maternal speech)
  figurative language, 30, 32
  function words, 15
  gestural communication, early, 102-103
  grammatical constructions, 15-16, 22
  illocutionary acts, 26-27
  imitation, 5-6, 17 (*see also* Imitation)
  indices, 43, 45, 52
  investigative trends, 101
  learning styles, 7, 11
  lexicon (*see* Lexicon)

RJ 496 .L35 L362   132268

Language disorders in
 children /

DISCARDED BY

MACPHÁIDÍN LIBRARY

DATE DUE

Returned	Returned	
MAR 3 1 1998	Returned	
Returned	Returned	APR 1 4 2004
APR 2 8 1999	JUN 0 1 1998	
	FEB 2 8 '98	
APR 0 8 1994	Returned	
	4-1-98	
	Returned	
NOV 1 8 1994		
Returned		
	APR 2 6 2002	MAY 1 4 2004
Returned	MAY 1 1 2007	
DEC 0 1 199	NOV 1 4 2007	
Returned		
MAR turned 97		

CUSHING-MARTIN LIBRARY
STONEHILL COLLEGE
NORTH EASTON, MASSACHUSETTS 02356